EMT EXAM PREP

FIFTH EDITION

S

© 2021 Kaplan

Published by Kaplan Publishing, a division of Kaplan, Inc.
750 Third Avenue
New York, NY 10017

Printed in the United States of America

10 9 8 7 6 5 4 3 2 1

ISBN-13: 978-1-5062-7943-5

Kaplan Publishing books are available at special quantity discounts to use for sales promotions, employee premiums, or educational purposes. For more information or to purchase books, please call the Simon & Schuster special sales department at 866-506-1949.

TABLE OF CONTENTS

For Test Changes or Late-Breaking Developments

kaptest.com/publishing

The material in this book is up-to-date at the time of publication. However, changes in the test may have been instituted after this book was published. Be sure to carefully read the materials you receive when you register for the test. If there are any important late-breaking developments—or any changes or corrections to the Kaplan test preparation materials in this book—we will post that information online at **kaptest.com/publishing**.

About the Author

Jessica Edwards, NRP, has been in the emergency services field for 15 years, starting off as an EMT for 10 years before moving forward to become a paramedic. Working in places such as Pennsylvania, Arizona, and even Israel, she is currently a cruise ship paramedic sailing around the world. Her interest in emergency services began in 2005, when she joined a volunteer fire department. She hasn't looked back, and hopes that her career will continue to be the adventure it has been thus far.

Since 2010, she has become an EMS instructor, an American Heart Association instructor for multiple disciplines, and a senior lead instructor for the EMT-Basic class at Gateway Community College in Phoenix, AZ.

Previous contributions by **Richard J. Lapierre**, MA,
EMT-Cardiac Director (Ret) of Brown University EMS

How to Use This Book

The book you have in front of you is not designed to reteach you the EMT curriculum, as you should have already successfully passed that portion of your path already. It is instead designed to refresh and review key elements that are commonly asked on the cognitive portion of the National Registry cognitive (knowledge) exam (NREMT).

By reading the chapters and taking the many practice questions and tests, at the end of the text you should feel confident in your ability to pass the exam.

The emergency services is a profession where you may not always receive a thank you, but you may get to see people at possibly the worst or best moments of their lives. Our contact may be for a few minutes at a time, but what you choose to do in those moments will have a real impact on someone's overall care.

So, study hard and realize that you're not just studying to pass an exam, you are also going to be part of the medical care of another human being and have the potential to change people's lives.

STEP 1: FAMILIARIZE YOURSELF WITH THE EXAM.

The first chapter of this book covers the basics, from the subjects that typically appear on the exam to administration and scoring. This section is designed to ease your anxiety about what appears on the exam.

STEP 2: REVIEW THE CONTENT CHAPTERS, PAYING SPECIAL ATTENTION TO ANY WEAK AREAS.

- Using the topic list at the start of each chapter, review the content areas one by one. Focus on items that you feel challenging.
- Do the "Test Yourself" exercises throughout the book and then check the answers at the back.
- Finally, do the Practice Sets at the end of each chapter. Read the explanations carefully to reinforce the material, especially those for any questions you got wrong.

STEP 3: CONCLUDE WITH THE EMT PRACTICE TEST, WHICH COVERS THE CONCEPTS TESTED ON THE EXAM.

After completing this exam, work through the explanations that follow it. Be sure to review the explanations for questions you got right as well as for those you got wrong. This will serve as a good review of the wide range of topics covered on the exam.

It is recommended you try to take the test all in one sitting with no breaks. Set a timer for 2 hours and attempt to finish the exam in this amount of time. This will prepare you for what it is like on Test Day and get you in the right mind-frame for when you are under a time limit.

STEP 4: STUDY A LITTLE BIT EVERY DAY BEFORE THE EXAM.

This is especially important if you schedule the exam weeks or even months in advance. Once you have finished your course, it is critical to remain current on the topics you have learned.

With consistency and focused study, you should achieve your goal of becoming a practicing EMT. Good luck!

The Basics

CHAPTER 1

Inside the EMT Cognitive Exam

Topics Discussed

- The Certification Process
- The Layout of the National Registry Exam
- The CAT Exam Structure
- What to Expect on Test Day

Congratulations on your decision to become an emergency medical technician (EMT). While you haven't chosen an easy profession, it is an important and essential one—one that earns the respect of the communities you serve. While no one really wants to need your services, you will be one of the most welcome sights in any emergency.

In the field of emergency medical services (EMS), there are various levels of certification:

- **EMT-Basic (most common)**
  - Entry-level patient care provider
  - Also called **EMT** or **BLS** (Basic Life Support)
  - Often used as a first step in career development for becoming a paramedic, firefighter, doctor, or nurse
  - Most limited scope of practice
- **EMT-Intermediate or Advanced** (EMT-I or EMT-A)
  - Currently, the NREMT only has advanced certification (intermediate level has been phased out, but those who already have EMT-I certification can convert their certification).
  - More expansive in scope of practice: can begin IVs, perform EKGs, give some medications (often including certain narcotics for pain management), and use airway adjuncts such as a laryngeal mask (LMA), which sits above the epiglottis.
- **Paramedics**
  - Also called **ALS** (Advanced Life Support) or medics (but their official lettering scheme is EMT-P or NRP for Nationally Registered Paramedic).
  - Highest level of certification in EMS, but there are specialties one may pursue such as flight or critical care level. These require additional schooling and certification.

– Broadest scope of practice that includes but is not limited to airway intubation, starting and maintaining IVs, administering more than 30 different medications for various conditions, performing and interpreting EKGs, and many others.

The main difference between an EMT and a paramedic is that the paramedic has more advanced training and a broader scope of practice. For example:

- An **EMT** can perform CPR and utilize an AED for persons in cardiac arrest.
- An **EMT** can provide basic oxygen or assist with a prescribed inhaler for those with difficulty breathing.
- An **EMT** cannot provide treatment that involves invasive measures into the body, e.g., an IV. (Certain procedures are allowed in some states, e.g., providing an airway that goes beyond the back of the tongue.)
- A **paramedic** is an advanced provider of emergency medical care whose work involves advanced resuscitation of patients beyond using an AED and compressions, including injecting IV medications and providing advanced airway assistance to patients.

Becoming an EMT-Basic

Not everyone can become an EMT. In addition to the proper frame of mind and desire, there are also educational and physical standards. Whether you are a state-certified EMT or a nationally registered EMT, the certification process pathway has three required steps:

- Successfully complete a state-approved EMT course (150–300 hours)
- Pass a psychomotor exam (physical, hands-on knowledge)
- Pass a cognitive exam (computer-based knowledge)

Once all of the components have been completed and passed, only then can the student become a registered practitioner.

State Certification: A few states **do not require** NREMT certification as their initial pathway to becoming a practitioner. (As of this printing, those states are Montana, Alaska, Illinois, New York, and North Carolina.) If you live in one of those states, you must follow the requirements by the state EMS office to gain your initial certification. However, it will closely follow the three steps listed above.

One downside to being only state-certified is that if you wish to move to a different state that requires NREMT certification you may be required to do additional testing. That is one of the main benefits of being an NREMT—it makes transferring certification much easier in the long run.

NREMT Certification: As of this printing, 45 states in the United States require EMT candidates to get initial certification through the National Registry of Emergency Medical Technicians (NREMT). In order to become a nationally registered EMT, you must have successfully completed the following steps/courses:

- State-approved EMT course that meets or exceeds National Emergency Medical Services Education Standards for the Emergency Medical Technician
  - Course must have been completed within previous 2 years
  - Program director must verify course completion on the NREMT website
- National Registry cognitive (knowledge) and state-approved psychomotor (skills) exams (passed portions remain valid for 24 months)
- CPR-BLS for "Healthcare Provider" or equivalent credential

The purpose of this book is to prepare you for the **National Registry cognitive (knowledge) exam** (NREMT).

Also, for the remainder of this book, whenever it states the letters EMT, it is always in reference to what is known longhand as EMT-Basic. It is true that a paramedic is also known as an EMT-P, however in everyday language, they are known as *paramedics* or just *medics*. It is understood that **when another EMS personnel states "EMT," that is referencing someone who is certified at the Basic level**.

Passing the Cognitive Exam

Exam Structure

The NREMT cognitive exam is a computer-based standardized test designed to measure your competence. The questions are written by a committee made up of EMS providers and other health and educational personnel; test scores are constantly monitored to assure accuracy and fairness.

The exam uses the computer-adaptive testing (CAT) method, which allows you to progress to more difficult questions as you answer previous questions correctly. Once the test ascertains that you are competent in a particular area, it moves on to the next.

Registration: To apply for the NREMT exam, go to **www.nremt.org**. You can register and pay online, and after training and state verification can schedule your exam through the NREMT website. Testing sites are available in most states.

As of this printing, the fee for the EMT exam is $80, which covers both the registration fee and testing center cost (regardless of test location).

Exam format

- You will have 2 hours to complete the exam.
- There will be 70–120 multiple-choice questions, many of which are scenario-based.
- There are five content areas (80% on patient care of adults; 20% on patient care of children):

  1. **Airway, Respiration, and Ventilation**: 18–22% of exam
  2. **Cardiology and Resuscitation**: 20–24% of exam
  3. **Medical; Obstetrics and Gynecology**: 27–31% of exam
  4. **Trauma**: 14–18% of exam
  5. **EMS Operations**: 10–14% of exam

The format of the exam is a **computerized-adaptive test (CAT)**, a type of computer-based test that adapts to each test taker's ability. Instead of having a predetermined mix of basic, medium, and hard questions, the computer selects questions based on how well you are doing, i.e., how well you are answering the previous questions. You will see only one question at a time.

In other words, every test taker takes a unique test, i.e., no two tests are alike.

- If you keep answering the questions correctly, the exam will get harder.
- If you answer some questions incorrectly, the exam will start to give you easier questions. If you get those easier questions right, it will pick up again giving you harder ones.
- You cannot return to a question once you've answered it or skip around within a section, because that would throw off the sequence. Once you answer a question, it's part of your score—for better or worse.

Using certain CAT-specific strategies can have a direct, positive impact on your score:

- Use the computer tutorial to your advantage. Spend as much time as you need to make yourself comfortable with the computer before you begin. If you click on Help once the exam is under way, it will count against your allotted time for that section.
- The CAT does not begin with really easy questions that gradually get harder. Because the order of difficulty will not be predictable, always be on the lookout for traps.
- A key strategy for doing well on the CAT is to perform well early on so that you quickly get to the point where you're being given the hard questions. Getting a hard question right will help your score a lot, but getting a hard question wrong will hurt your score only slightly. Thus, it pays to spend more time on those early questions, double-checking each answer before you confirm it.
- Try to avoid getting several questions in a row wrong. If the previous question you answered was a blind guess, spend a little extra time on the next question.
- The CAT does not allow you to go back to questions you've already answered to double-check your work, so be as certain as possible that you have answered a question correctly before moving on.

- The CAT does not allow you to skip questions. So, if you are given a question you cannot answer, you'll have to guess. Eliminate any wrong answer choices that you can spot and guess intelligently and strategically among those remaining.

- Sometimes it's necessary to give up on a tough, time-consuming question. It's difficult to do, but let it go and move on to the next question. That's how you score points—not by agonizing over one question.

- Don't get rattled if you keep seeing really, really difficult questions. It just means you're doing very well on that section. Keep it up!

A CAT exam is structurally different from a paper-and-pencil exam. In a CAT, it is not the **number of questions** answered that determines whether you pass, but rather the **difficulty of questions** (and your answers). Someone may pass having answered 72 questions, while another person may fail having answered 72 questions.

Scoring

- You will receive a **pass or fail** score, not a numerical score.

- Students who pass will receive a congratulatory message with a link to the official certification card. Passing the exam means you are a certified EMT, able to perform the procedures for which you have been trained in your state.

- Students who do not pass will receive a breakdown of specific "weak areas," e.g., airway or medical emergencies, so they can focus their study for a second attempt.

Exam Strategies

Since this test is such an important milestone in an EMT's career, good test-taking skills are crucial. To succeed, you've got to get enough right answers in each section of the test. Knowing the material is not enough. You have to perfect your mindset and time-management skills so that you get a chance to use your knowledge on as many questions as possible.

It's one thing to answer one question correctly; it's quite another to answer up to 120 of them in 120 minutes and get more than 70% right. And the same goes for those long scenario questions—it's a whole new ball game once you move from doing individual practice at your leisure to handling dozens of questions under timed conditions.

So, when you're comfortable with the content of the test, your next challenge will be to take it to the next level—test expertise—which will enable you to manage the all-important time element of the test.

Use Process of Elimination for the Answers

Using a process of elimination is a way to answer questions both quickly and effectively. There are two ways to get all the answers right on the exam: you know all the right answers, or you know all the wrong answers. Since there are three times as many wrong answers, you should be able to eliminate some, if not all, of them. By doing so, you either get to the correct response or increase your chances of guessing the correct response.

You start out with a 25% chance of selecting the right answer, and with each eliminated answer choice your odds go up. Eliminate one, and you'll have a 33% chance of picking the right one; eliminate two, and you'll have a 50% chance, etc.

Remember to look for wrong-answer traps when you're eliminating. Some answer choices are designed to distract you by distorting the correct answer.

Remain Calm and Keep Track of Time

It's imperative to remain calm and composed while working through the test. You can't allow yourself to become so rattled by one hard question that it throws you off. Keep these thoughts in mind when you face a tough question:

- Having trouble with a tough question won't ruin your score—but getting upset about it and letting it throw you off track will.
- When you understand that part of the test maker's goal is to reward those who keep their composure, you'll recognize the importance of not panicking when you run into challenging material.

At the same time, you can't let yourself run out of time. It's essential to pace yourself, keeping in mind the general guidelines for how long to spend on any individual question (a bit less than 1 minute). Don't spend a wildly disproportionate amount of time on any one question.

Be Aware of What's Needed on the Test

This test is like no other test you've taken before. If you took a test in high school or college and got a number of the questions wrong, you wouldn't receive a perfect grade. But on this test, you can get a number of questions wrong and still get a "perfect" passing score.

- The test is geared so that only the very best test takers are able to answer every question. But even these people rarely get every question right.
- What does that mean for you? For starters, don't let what you consider to be a subpar performance on one or two questions ruin your performance on the entire test. If you allow that subpar performance to rattle you, it can have a cumulative negative effect, setting in motion a downward spiral. It's that kind of thing that could potentially do serious damage to your score.
- Losing a few extra points won't do you in, but losing your cool will.

Remember, if you feel you've done poorly on a scenario, even one with more than one related question, don't sweat it. Remain calm and collected and simply do your best.

Build Stamina and Confidence

You must work on your test-taking stamina, as the exam is long and fairly challenging. Additionally, you must build up your confidence, which will lead to quick, sure answers and a sense of well-being that translates into more points.

- Take the full-length practice test included in this book. You'll be able to review answer explanations and assess your performance. Be sure to go over your wrong answers.
- If you lack confidence you end up reading the sentences and answer choices two, three, and even four times, until you confuse yourself and get off track. This leads to timing difficulties, which only perpetuate the downward spiral, causing anxiety and a tendency to rush.

- Focus all of your practice on the major goal of taking control of the test. When you've achieved that goal—armed with the principles, techniques, strategies, and approaches set forth in this book—you'll be ready to face the exam with supreme confidence.

Have the Right Attitude

Don't waste time making value judgments about the exam. It's not going to go away. Those who look forward to doing battle with exams tend to score better than do those who resent or dread it.

It may sound a little dubious, but take our word for it: attitude adjustment is a proven test-taking technique.

- Look at the exam as a challenge, but try not to obsess over it; you certainly don't want to psych yourself out of the game.

- Yes, the exam is obviously important, but, contrary to what some candidates think, this one test will not single-handedly determine the outcome of your life.

- Try to have fun with the exam! Learning how to match your wits against the test makers can be a very satisfying experience, and the reading and thinking skills you'll acquire will benefit you in the EMS.

- Remember that you're more prepared than most people. You've trained with Kaplan. You have the tools you need, plus the know-how to use those tools.

On Test Day

It should go without saying that on the day of the test you should prepare by being totally rested and focused on the task at hand. Cramming at the last minute by going over your notes will not achieve the desired result if you haven't been studying them all along. Pulling an all-nighter a day or two in advance of Test Day will also be counterproductive (plus, you run the risk of falling asleep during the exam).

Here are some pointers:

- Arrive at the test site at least 30 minutes before the announced start time. This will give you time to collect your thoughts instead of rushing in to take the exam.

- Do not bring your notes with you, as at this point they will be more of a distraction than anything else. And they are not allowed in the test!

- Most testing sites will either give you paper and pen or an erasable writing board to have during the exam. While you may use it however you like during the exam, you may not take this with you when you leave.

- Some testing sites do not allow food or water, so eat and drink before the exam accordingly.

- If you start to feel distracted, overwhelmed, or tired, stop. Close your eyes, and try to clear your mind. Eat some of your snack and drink some water. Take a few deep breaths and then continue. If this doesn't clear your mind sufficiently, the proctor will have given directions as to using the restroom. Usually no more than one person at a time is permitted to leave. If you can do so, go to the restroom and splash water on your face. All of this will help you refocus to the task at hand.

- Keep an eye on the clock, as you do not want to run out of time.

- If you cannot answer a question with certainty, analyze it and give it your best guess. You will not be allowed to move on to the next question without answering the previous question.

EMT Review

CHAPTER 2

Well-Being of the EMT

Topics Discussed

- **Physical, Emotional, and Mental Risks Posed to the EMT**
- **Types of Patient Consent to Treatment**
- **How the Law Protects the Medical Provider**
- **Management of Crime Scenes as a Medical Provider**

Prehospital emergency medicine is a tough, demanding practice. It requires not only physical strength and conditioning, but mental and emotional stability as well.

To be able to go from a relaxed state of mind to one where you will have to potentially make critical decisions in moments at any hour of the day involves the entire being. This chapter will discuss the many risks that EMTs face at any given time (on the job or off duty): physical, mental, and emotional.

Risks of the Job

Physical Risks

The most obvious danger to an EMT's well-being is physical danger. Physical danger can present in various ways: personal threats, environmental hazards (chemical spills, building collapses), and communicable disease (hepatitis, SARS).

The following are set as per national EMS operating guidelines:

- As an EMT you are not allowed to enter any scene you believe to be dangerous or presents a personal threat (e.g., a patient with a weapon). That type of scenario must be secured by law enforcement prior to your entry. Do not attempt to disarm anyone holding a weapon. Call for police backup or defer to the police if they are already on scene.
- As an EMT you must be aware of the dangers of bloodborne and airborne pathogens, know how to prevent contamination, and know how to handle articles exposed to bodily fluids that may be contaminated. Exposure to communicable diseases such as hepatitis, tuberculosis, and HIV is preventable with inoculation and the use of protective devices (masks, gloves).

- The proper use and disposal of hypodermic needles and syringes (often called "sharps") is paramount. One of the most common causes of prehospital exposure to pathogens among EMTs is the "dirty needle stick." These are mostly preventable with proper use and disposal techniques.

While heroics are common in the movies, the reality is that entry into an unsafe scene has the potential to cause you harm, which would complicate the response. It would also prevent you from being able to assist on the initial call.

Mental and Emotional Risks

In addition to the physical danger, there is also the emotional trauma of being an EMT. Many EMS professionals can tell you that they have had at least one really tough call that has stuck with them to this day. For longevity in this career, the emotionally healthy EMT takes this trauma, processes it (with counseling if needed), and moves forward.

The formal response to this type of trauma may be a critical incident stress debriefing (CISD). These are conducted formally by other public safety personnel within 24 to 72 hours following a critical incident and may be followed up with a recommendation for some formal type of one-on-one intervention.

While every EMT has wanted to resuscitate an apneic and pulseless patient, the fact is that death and dying are part of this profession: In her book *On Death and Dying*, Dr. Elisabeth Kubler-Ross clarifies five stages in dealing with death: denial and isolation, anger, bargaining, depression, and acceptance. These stages hold true for both the family members of the deceased and also the EMS providers on the scene.

Many people entering the ranks of prehospital emergency medicine are young adults whose experiences with death may be very limited. It is important for their mentors and officers to recognize the signs of post-traumatic stress disorder (PTSD) and be prepared to intervene and assist as needed.

Substance Abuse

Unfortunately, some EMS providers fall prey to using substances such as alcohol or illicit drugs in order to cope with the stress of the profession. This is not said to scare you or anyone away from becoming an EMT, but it is worth saying that we must collectively look after our own well-being as well as our partner's, as someone may be struggling and no one will know until it's too late.

If you or someone you know is struggling with substance abuse, please know that it is okay to reach out and ask for help. Many companies provide access to an employee assistance program (EAP), which can recommend and help coordinate treatment for many situations, including substance abuse. Consulting and treatment will remain confidential. However, providers must be aware that each company has the right to randomly drug test any provider they hire as a condition of employment. They expect providers to be of clear mind and body in order to serve the public they have in their coverage area, so there is often a strict no-drugs policy that can result in termination or legal implications.

Post-Traumatic Stress Disorder

Post-traumatic stress disorder (PTSD) is an anxiety disorder that can develop after experiencing a shocking or dangerous event, such as war or trauma. Symptoms usually arise within 3 months of the event but sometimes can take years to manifest. Various studies show that 20–55% of EMS providers will experience PTSD symptoms or are formally diagnosed with the disorder.

The signs and symptoms of PTSD include the following:

- Unexplained irritability
- Inability to concentrate or make decisions
- Difficulty sleeping, nightmares
- Anxiety
- Feelings of guilt
- Loss of appetite, sexual desire, interest in work
- Possible suicidal thoughts (in an effort to stop feeling any of the emotions above)

Any symptoms that persist for longer than a few days should be considered serious. Anyone experiencing these symptoms in themselves or witnessing them in coworkers should notify their superior immediately so that the situation may be dealt with either within the service or referred to a competent outside provider.

A good defense against serious PTSD is the sharing of one's emotions in confidence with one's coworkers, especially those who were part of the call and are familiar with the details, or with those who have been through something similar on other calls. Depending on the severity of the call, processing these emotions may take months or even years.

Medical, Legal, and Ethical Issues

As an EMT, the particular state and service protocols under which you function will determine your scope of practice and standard of care. These protocols are the legal framework under which patient care is guided, so it is imperative that you know them well. Furthermore, deviating from these protocols could result in impaired treatment and/or legal action.

Duty to Act

While the application of the rule varies from state to state, the duty to act is a legal requirement to take action that will prevent harm to another person or the general public. In the context of EMS providers, this means responding to calls in a rapid but safe manner, performing a thorough assessment, administering the necessary treatment, and transporting to a receiving facility when needed.

Legally, the EMT is bound by the following conditions:

- If an EMT is **on duty** as a prehospital medical provider, he has a duty to act on any ill or injured patient that is encountered or dispatched to. It is not permissible to refuse an intervention, regardless of personal preference.

- If an EMT is **off duty** and encounters an ill or injured person, he may feel an ethical duty to assist, but there is no mandate to do so. While wanting to assist is an admirable trait, use caution when deciding to proceed, as liability coverage is usually very limited under these circumstances. This is not to discourage you from helping someone during leisure time, but be aware of the risks.

Patient Consent

The issue of patient consent is one of the trickiest of all medical, legal, and ethical issues. It is a generally accepted legal principle that a competent individual has the right to permit or refuse any specific medical procedure.

A common example is when the EMT is confronted with a victim of a motor vehicle accident who refuses to allow the application of a cervical collar, which many states require of all trauma victims with a possibility of cervical trauma. Thus, the EMT now is faced with two conflicting ideas. The competent person's right of refusal will normally take precedence; however, it has been argued that a reasonable and prudent person would want the collar, and thus collars have been forced upon patients. The EMT has to be aware that such an action may well be considered assault and battery should the patient choose to file a lawsuit.

- **Expressed consent** is verbal agreement to treatment by a competent patient.
- **Implied consent** means a patient who is unconscious, inebriated, or otherwise unable to express consent would agree to treatment as would be given to anyone in that situation.
- *In loco parentis* is a specialized term that is used for underage or pediatric patients whose parents/guardians are not present but would reasonably agree to treatment of their child in an emergency situation. It translates to "in the place of parents."

TEST YOURSELF 2.1

What type of consent is this?

A school nurse calls 911 for a child experiencing anaphylactic shock. The child has never had a prescription for an epinephrine pen. The parents were called right away, but they have not yet responded. The child is experiencing severe respiratory distress with hives present. What is the EMT able to do?

Competency

When it comes to patient care, the word **competent** can also cause a dilemma in the emergency medical profession. It is a recognized legal fact that a person who is seriously intoxicated is not a competent person; however, there is no magic standard that defines the level of inebriation that creates incompetence. The EMT is thus thrust into the position of making this important determination on the scene and setting the level of medical care.

By utilizing various patient assessment tools such as the AVPU or alert and oriented scale or by speaking with medical command, the EMT can make the decision of whether or not a patient would be considered a competent person who could make reasonable decisions about the care they receive or refuse.

A minor is held by most states to lack competence, so even if a 9-year-old bicycle-accident victim refuses a cervical collar, the EMT can overrule that preference unless there is a parent on the scene who objects.

Litigation and the Good Samaritan Law

It is important for the EMT to know how legal defenses are handled with respect to performance of duties.

- When **off-duty,** the EMT is protected by the Good Samaritan Law, which provides immunity against liability for someone who performs an emergency medical procedure for which they are trained/licensed/certified, unless it is done in a grossly negligent manner. (*Negligence* is defined as "failure to use reasonable care, resulting in damage or injury to another.") In order to be successfully sued, lawyers must be able to prove that the person's actions caused damage/injury to the patient.
  - Suppose an EMT is certified in CPR and use of an AED, meaning she has been trained to use the hands placed on the lower half of the sternum, pushing down to a depth of 2-2.4 inches at a rate of 100-120 compressions per minute (current AHA standards).
  - If EMT chose instead to start compressions with the foot on the victim's chest or to not use a nearby AED, that could be considered grossly negligent.
- When **on-duty,** the EMT has a duty to act and follow protocols which in themselves provide a level of legal protection. *Medical direction* is one of those protocols.
  - With **online medical control,** the EMT communicates with an "online" emergency room physician to understand how to proceed with treatment.
  - With **offline medical control** (if online control cannot or does not need to be established), the EMT uses prior knowledge and standard protocols to decide how to proceed with treatment.

Confidentiality

Numerous laws and court decisions have assured the confidentiality of medical information. What is told to the EMT by a patient is confidential and is to be told only to those to whom the EMT transfers patient care.

The passage of the Health Insurance Portability and Accountability Act (HIPAA) in 1996 secured the legal requirement by all health care professionals to confidentially handle protected health information. As such, the EMT is bound by these requirements. It is never permissible to discuss a patient's history or care with anyone outside the medical community, unless compelled to do so by a legal order.

In the field, keeping the HIPAA confidentiality requirements poses certain challenges. EMT assessments are routinely carried out in a public setting, rather than a closed office. Someone is less likely to divulge a history of a sexually transmitted disease if there are coworkers standing nearby.

Legally speaking, however, there is certain information that a patient will provide during the course of your assessment that is considered to be protected health information (PHI).

- Assure the patient that everything is said in confidentiality, and that only those in their direct care will have access to their answers. (Some services have this information in writing, so this can be handed to the patient.)
- While this information is often needed to fill out your PCR and allow the company to appropriately bill for services, the patient has the right to "not answer" these questions.

The following information is considered PHI and should not be revealed to anyone outside of the patient's care.

- First or last name
- Address or phone number
- Social Security number or other identification number
- Date of birth
- Medical record number

While it may be hard to keep track of the various pieces of PHI, they are important to remember when writing your patient care report or giving a radio report.

Extreme care must be taken to protect the patient's identity.

Crime Scenes

When a medical scene is also a crime scene, care must be taken to disturb as little as possible. Documentation of patient care must also include any disturbances that were needed for the patient's treatment and transport.

Various state laws also address when medical personnel *must* notify law enforcement officials if they become aware of certain situations. If an EMT is aware that a child has been physically, emotionally, or sexually abused, failure to notify the proper agency may subject the EMT not only to civil but to criminal penalties as well.

- If you suspect the abuse of a person or have identified physical indicators of such, you must document it in your patient care report and also let the receiving medical team know of your observations or suspicions.

- It is better to let the proper personnel know and have it turn out to be a false alarm, versus to say nothing and run the risk of further harm taking place later.

- Remember it is the EMT's duty to perform both medical care and patient advocacy.

Some states also provide for the notification of sudden death, overdoses of illicit drugs, gunshot wounds, spousal abuse, sexual abuse, elder abuse, and animal bites. Please follow your local or state protocols to make sure you are aware of when and whom to notify of such situations.

EMS falls under what is typically called a "mandated reporter," i.e., emergency personnel are responsible for notifying the proper authorities if there is suspected abuse of vulnerable populations, particularly children.

Practice Set

1. You are dispatched to a call for a possible overdose. You are advised that police response will be delayed. Upon arrival on scene, you are directed to a bedroom at the end of a hall. Opening the door, you see a middle-aged female sitting on a bed, surrounded by open pill bottles and an empty whiskey bottle. She is waving around a large butcher knife. Which of the following is the correct course of action?

   A. Rush her and take the knife away from her

   B. Have your partner distract her while you take the knife away

   C. Withdraw from the room to a position of safety and request that police expedite their response

   D. Talk her into giving you the knife

2. You and your partner respond to a call involving the death of an infant. The following week, your partner tells you that he has been having nightmares involving the death of his own children and that he is not eating or sleeping well. Which of the following should be your next course of action?

   A. Slap him and tell him to snap out of it

   B. Notify your immediate supervisor of your concerns

   C. Do nothing

   D. Drive him immediately to the nearest mental health facility

3. You are called to the scene of a man down with no other information. You arrive on scene, and your partner quickly assesses the patient, turns to you, and shakes his head. The patient is cyanotic with full rigor and postmortem-dependent lividity clearly present in his torso. The man's wife is anxious, peering into the room and asking you if he will be all right. You gently lead her into the living room and ask her to sit down. Looking directly at her, you quietly say that her husband has died and there is nothing that you can do. She initially has no reaction, then wails loudly and throws herself into your arms, crying out, "He can't be dead; he was just talking to me!" What is this stage of grief called?

   A. Acceptance

   B. Bargaining

   C. Anger

   D. Denial

4. After discharging a patient who had been stabbed in the abdomen to the emergency department, you are removing your bloody gloves when you notice that they are torn and blood has gotten on your skin. Furthermore, after you wash the blood off, you notice that you have a small, fresh laceration on your middle finger. What is your next course of action?

   A. Wash your hands again and that will take care of any contamination issues

   B. Disinfect the wound with hydrogen peroxide and dress it with a sterile dressing

   C. Use alcohol hand sanitizer to wash the laceration

   D. Report a bloodborne-pathogen exposure to your immediate supervisor and follow your service's protocol for exposure

5. Which of the following situations violates a person's protected health information (PHI)?

   A. Documenting your patient's full name in your patient care report and submitting it to your service for billing

   B. Verifying through your lawyer that you treated a patient after being subpoenaed for a lawsuit concerning that particular person in question

   C. Attaching a copy of the patient's hospital information sheet to your patient care report for billing purposes

   D. Stating the patient's full name and your estimated arrival time while giving a prehospital radio report to the receiving hospital

6. You arrive on the scene of a "man down" call. Upon arrival you observe a male in his mid-forties, lying face up on the sidewalk. He is snoring and you smell what you believe to be an alcoholic beverage on his breath. What legal doctrine allows you to begin treatment since he does not respond to your verbal questioning?

   A. Good Samaritan Act

   B. *In loco parentis*

   C. Implied consent

   D. Expressed consent

7. You are dispatched to an unknown-type medical call. You respond emergently and arrive at a residence. Police have secured the scene, and when you enter the apartment you see a male in his fifties lying on a couch. He is semi-conscious and smells of liquor. His response to your questioning is belligerent, and he repeatedly asks you to leave him alone and tells you that he is fine. He is unable to tell you what day it is or where he currently is. His breathing is rapid and shallow, and he appears to be pale and diaphoretic. What is your next course of action?

   A. Have the patient sign a refusal form and go back in service

   B. Advise the patient that he may be seriously ill and continue to encourage him to allow you to transport him to a medical facility

   C. Drag the patient off the couch, have the police put him in handcuffs, and march him out to your truck for transport

   D. Advise the police that due to his medical condition, the patient must be transported and may not refuse due to incompetence because of suspected alcohol intoxication, and request that they assist you in placing the subject in the truck

Answers and Explanations

1. C

When faced with this situation, the other solutions appear to be more heroic; however, all other answers involve the EMT placing themselves at risk to be injured.

2. B

Your partner is exhibiting symptoms of depression and anxiety brought on by post-traumatic stress. While nothing here suggests that the stress is critical at this time, you have a duty to act and seek proper care for him. Notify your supervisor of your concerns so that proper mental health care can be obtained. The "snap out of it" approach only works well in the movies. Doing nothing may allow the situation to resolve itself, but it also may allow your partner to slip into a clinical depression. Driving him to the mental health facility without having done a proper workup may be counterproductive and could damage your relationship.

3. D

Denial is a common first reaction to difficult news: "If I don't believe it, it didn't really happen." News of tragic importance is often accompanied by a wide range of emotions, as the mind attempts to absorb information it doesn't really want to hear. As such, the mind will process the emotions with whatever "controls" it can find to try and delay the final stage of grief (acceptance). Anger may also be the first stage and the EMT often bears the brunt of the attack, both verbal and physical: "They always save the patient on television, what did you do wrong?" Know that an angry response is a defense mechanism. Bargaining serves the same purpose.

4. D

The combination of skin exposure to someone else's blood and an open wound could mean that bloodborne pathogens have been introduced into your bloodstream. These pathogens can include HIV and hepatitis, both of which can cause serious illnesses and are potentially fatal. (A), (B), and (C) deal with external exposure and will not be effective if the pathogen has already been introduced into the bloodstream. Each service is

required by law to have a protocol for these exposures, which includes blood testing and medical consultation for treatments to minimize the risk of developing blood-borne illnesses; however, this is only effective if implemented and the appropriate personnel are notified.

5. D

While prehospital radio reports may seem secure, they are in fact easily accessible by nonmedical personnel and can be heard by anyone who knows which frequency to tune in to. Revealing a patient's full name is not only *not required* to give a radio report, but it clearly identifies the patient to random individuals who have nothing to do with patient care. This is imperative for the EMT to remember at all times.

6. C

The correct answer is implied consent. The law allows the EMT (or any medical provider) to assume that the patient, if conscious, would consent to normal medical treatments. The Good Samaritan Act covers the EMT while off duty and not working in an official capacity at the time of incident. *In loco parentis* is the type of consent used in pediatric cases where the parents or guardian are not on scene but would reasonably give permission to treat their child. Expressed consent is when the patient consciously and competently gives you permission to perform a medical procedure.

7. D

The key is that the patient does not know what day it is or where he is. These factors give you the criteria you need to overrule his rejection of a transport, since he probably lacks the competence to refuse. (A) is only correct if you are satisfied that the patient will be fine if he signs a refusal and you leave. It is always good to remember that somebody felt concerned enough to call EMS, and you should be extremely cautious in accepting a refusal from a patient who is presenting with serious symptoms. (B) is not correct because the amount of time you should spend arguing with an intoxicated patient is limited. (C) is not part of your job description and is properly done by law enforcement.

CHAPTER 3

Anatomy and Physiology

Topics Discussed

- Anatomical Directions and Planes
- Musculoskeletal System
- Respiratory and Circulatory Systems
- Gastrointestinal System
- Genitourinary and Reproductive System
- Nervous, Integumentary, and Endocrine Systems

As a medical provider, the EMT must be familiar with the standard terminology of medical practice, including anatomical and physiological definitions. A good working knowledge of anatomy and physiology is necessary not only for the practice of prehospital medicine, but also for communication with other medical professionals.

A large portion of the EMT exam focuses on the pathophysiology of the various body systems and how they contribute to various illnesses or accidents a patient may experience. The EMT must have a basic understanding of organs and structures in order to properly identify treatments as well as pitfalls that may occur if a wrong treatment is administered.

Anatomical Terminology

In order to ensure that communication across health care is consistent, standard naming conventions are used to describe the locations and positions on the body. This is especially important for the EMT when assessing a patient, when communicating with the receiving hospital staff, and when writing a patient care report.

Planes

Anatomical planes are imaginary lines that divide the body into sections. Knowledge of planes allows the EMT to communicate important information about the injury to other medical personnel. The exam will include a variety of questions about directions and planes.

In practice, anatomical terms are patient-oriented, i.e., "right side" refers to the *patient's* right side.

Look at the graphic below and follow along with the labels to make sure you understand each term presented. For instance, using the options *proximal*, *distal*, *lateral*, or *medial*, which choice would be correct for "the thumb is _____ to the wrist"?

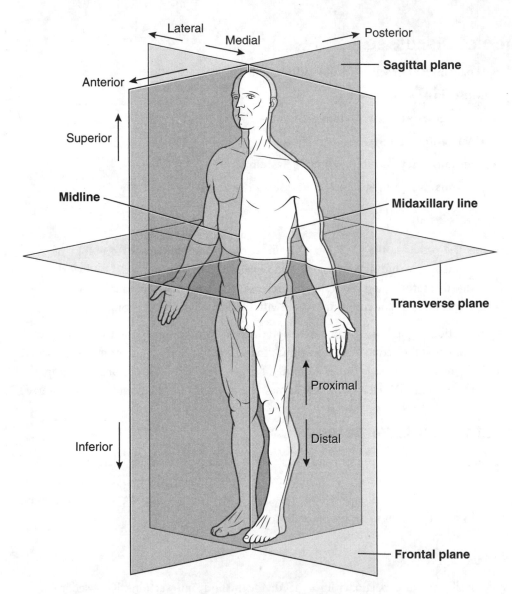

Figure 3.1 *Anatomical Planes*

Terms Explained

Anatomical and directional terms help to clarify where one body part is in relation to another.

Table 3.1 *Anatomical Terms*

Terminology	Definition	Example
Anatomical position	Position where a person stands upright, with palms facing forward and thumbs facing away from the body	
Midline/sagittal plane • **Lateral** objects go away from the midline • **Medial** objects move toward the midline	Imaginary vertical line dividing the body into left and right side	• **Lateral:** the eye is lateral to the nose • **Medial:** the nose is medial to the ears
Midaxillary line/frontal plane • **Anterior** objects are on the front portion of the body • **Posterior** objects are on the back portion of the body • **Ventral:** toward the front of the torso • **Dorsal:** toward the back of the torso	Imaginary vertical line dividing the body into front and back portions	• **Anterior:** the nose is on the anterior portion of the head • **Posterior:** the gluteal muscles (buttocks) are located on the posterior • **Ventral:** the naval belly button is ventral to the lumbar spinal vertebrae • **Dorsal:** the shoulder blade is dorsal to the ribs
Transverse plane • **Superior:** meaning above or up • **Inferior:** meaning down or toward the bottom	Imaginary horizontal line dividing the body into top and bottom portions	• **Superior:** the head is superior to the feet • **Inferior:** the foot is inferior to the patella (knee)
Limbs • **Proximal** objects are closer to the torso • **Distal** objects are farther (distant) from the torso	Extensions from the torso (trunk of the body) that include the arms (connected via the shoulder) and the legs (connected via the hips)	• **Proximal:** the elbow is proximal to the wrist • **Distal:** the fingers are distal to the elbows

---

TEST YOURSELF 3.1

Can you locate the wound?

You are dispatched to a stabbing emergency. Upon arrival, you find a young male with a stab wound to the right thigh that is approximately 5 cm on the medial anterior side of the leg, proximal to the groin.

Picture the location in your head or draw on a piece of paper where the wound is located.

There are many other anatomical terms that describe movement of the limbs. In the next section, we'll break down the movements that can occur in each plane of the body.

Movements

Knowing how a limb moves within a certain plane of the body is immensely helpful for the EMT when trying to understand how an injury occurred or how to splint or bandage the affected part.

With the images below as your guide, use your own body to get a clear idea of the movements here. Think about what injury patterns could occur if these movements were interrupted or injured.

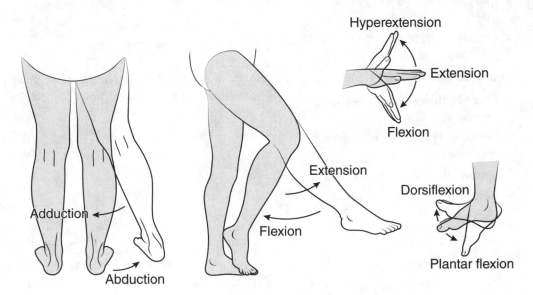

Figure 3.2 *Anatomical Movements*

Sagittal Plane: hyper ("more than") movements can occur in each section listed below.

- **Flexion**: decreasing the angle between two bones at a joint. Example is when you would bend your knee toward your body.
- **Extension**: increasing the angle between two bones at a joint. Example would be straightening the knee back out from a bent position.
- **Dorsiflexion** and **plantar flexion**: referring specifically to the foot, dorsiflexion is pointing the toes toward the head, while plantar flexion is pointing the sole of the foot toward the ground.

Frontal Plane

- **Adduction**: moving limb toward midline. A helpful reminder is that you "add" to the body. Example is moving your leg toward your other leg.

- **Abduction**: moving limb away from the midline. Think about how an abduction of something takes it away from somewhere or someone. Example is moving the leg away from the body as shown in the picture.

Transverse Plane

- **Rotation**: the movement that turns around the vertical axis of a bone. You can have internal (inward) or external (outward) motion. Example would be a hip fracture.

- **Pronation**: rotating a bone medially from another bone. Example would be when a person turns their feet toward the medial side of their body outward or "rolls" an ankle and feels pain.

- **Supination**: rotating a bone laterally from another bone. Picture turning your wrist so that you can hold a bowl of soup in your hand. Soup = supination.

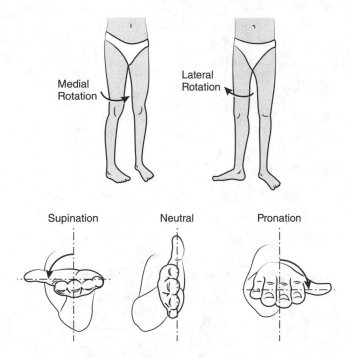

Figure 3.3 *Transverse Plane Movements*

Now let's move on to the individual body systems.

Musculoskeletal System

Skeletal System

The skeleton is a collection of bones that provides the framework of the human body. The bones also provide protection for the soft tissues and internal organs.

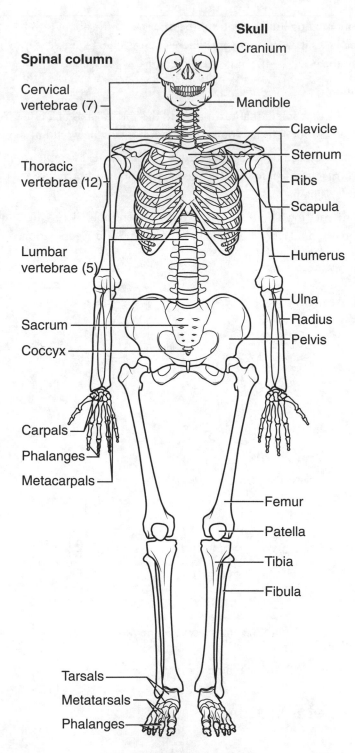

Figure 3.4 *Major Skeletal Bones*

The skeletal system is divided into seven sections: the skull, the face, the spinal column, the thorax, the pelvis, the upper extremities, and the lower extremities.

The **skull**—also known as the **cranium**—is a cap of bone that serves to protect the brain. Different sections of the skull make up the cap itself:

- **Frontal bone**: located where the forehead is
- **Parietal bones**: located on both sides of the head and above the ears; these span toward the back of the head where they meet with the occipital bone
- **Occipital bone**: located on the posterior portion of the head; protects the cerebellum region of the brain
- **Temporal bone**: located superior to the ear, on both sides of the head
- **Sphenoid bone**: located posterior from the orbital socket
- **Sutures**: fibrous bands of tissue that connect the bones of the skull together
- **Fontanelles** (found in pediatric patients): located anterior and posterior; where the sutures have not fully closed yet; typically close by age 18 months
- **Facial bones**: include the orbit (eye socket), nasal bone, maxilla and mandible (jaw), and zygomatic bones (cheeks)

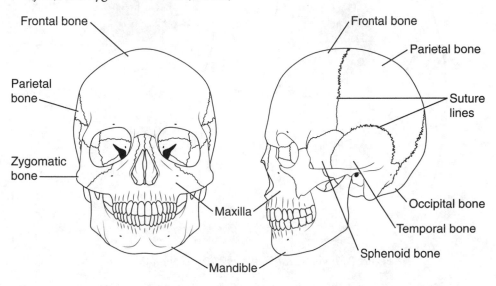

Figure 3.5 *Skull and Facial Bones*

Next, we have the **spinal column**, also known as the backbone. There are several sections of bones called the vertebrae, which are as follows:

- **Cervical** (aka neck) has seven vertebrae and is one of the most vulnerable portions of the spine due to its lack of protection from rest of the body.
- **Thoracic** (aka chest) has 12 vertebrae; the thorax or thoracic cavity is located here as well.
- **Lumbar** (aka low back) has five vertebrae; a lot of the body's load pressure is placed here and is a common location for pain complaints.
- **Sacral** (aka pelvis) is a set of five fused vertebrae; located within the pelvic cavity.
- **Coccyx** (aka tailbone) is a set of four fused vertebrae; it is susceptible to trauma.

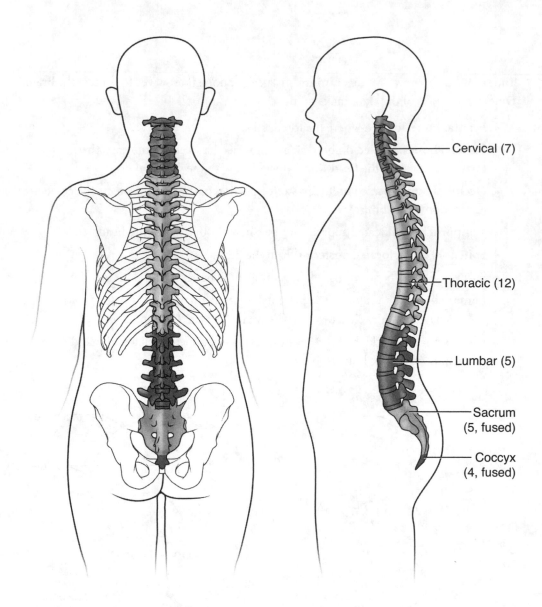

Figure 3.6 *Vertebral Sections of the Spinal Column*

On the exam, you are almost sure to be asked about the number of vertebrae composing a particular section of the spinal column.

The **thorax** or **chest cavity** is comprised of 12 pairs of ribs, 10 of which are connected to the sternum or breastbone.

- The bottom two ribs are called "floating ribs," since they are connected in the back to the vertebrae. They do not attach to the sternum or any other ribs.
- The space between the ribs is called **intercostal space**.
- The **sternum** is divided into three parts: the **manubrium** (or superior) portion, the middle body, and the **xiphoid process** (inferior tip).

The **pelvis** is located in the inferior portion of the abdominal cavity and protects the internal reproductive organs, intestines, bladder, and rectum. Its major bones are as follows:

- **Iliac crests**: the wing sections of the pelvis
- **Pubis**: the anterior portion of the pelvic bone
- **Ischium**: the inferior portion of the pelvis

Upper extremities (arms and shoulder girdle) are comprised of the following bones bilaterally:

- **Clavicle**: collarbone
- **Scapula**: shoulder blade
- **Humerus**: superior bone of the arm
- **Radius**: lateral bone of the forearm (the landmark is here for a radial pulse)
- **Ulna**: medial bone of the forearm (this is thumb side of the lower arm)
- **Carpals**: collective name of eight tiny bones that make up the wrist
- **Metacarpals**: collective name for the five bones of the hand
- **Phalanges**: finger bones

Lower extremities (**legs and pelvic girdle**) consist of the following bones bilaterally:

- **Greater trochanter** (ball) and **acetabulum** (socket): together form the hip joint
- **Femur**: thighbone
- **Patella**: kneecap
- **Tibia**: medial bone of the lower leg
- **Fibula**: lateral bone of the lower leg
- **Malleolus**: ankle bones on both medial and lateral sides
- **Tarsals** and **metatarsals**: 12 bones that make up the foot
- **Calcaneous**: heel of foot
- **Phalanges**: toe bones

Phalanges are in both the hand and the foot, so be specific about referencing their location.

Muscular System

Joints and Connections

A joint is where more than two bones connect. The basic joint types are **ball and socket** (hip and shoulder) and **hinge** (elbow and knee).

To facilitate movement at the joint, there are two special fibrous **connections** called tendons and ligaments.

- Bones are connected to muscles by tendons.
- Bones are connected to other bones by ligaments.

Both of these connections provide motion ability, such as being able to bend your arm at the elbow or lift your leg and bend at the hip.

Muscle Types

There are three types of muscle in the body, which give the skeletal system the ability to move, give the body its shape, and supply protection for the internal organs of the body. Muscles are also differentiated by whether they are **voluntary** (requiring conscious control) or **involuntary** (cannot be voluntarily controlled or willed).

- **Skeletal** muscle (**voluntary**) connects to the skeletal bones and allows them to move in various ways. Actions are controlled by the brain and nervous system.
- **Smooth** muscle (**mostly involuntary**) is under the control of the autonomic nervous system and functions as necessary for the body to exist.
  - The diaphragm, which controls lung inflation or deflation, will work no matter the will of the individual, but may temporarily be overridden by the person's conscious action, i.e., holding one's breath.
  - The digestive process muscles (e.g., esophagus and intestines) move the food particles along the path toward elimination and help the body absorb nutrients along the way.
- **Cardiac muscle** (involuntary but unique and classified by itself, due to its ability for automaticity, or the ability to generate electrical impulses on its own) allows the heart to pump blood to the rest of the body and is found only within the heart itself.

Respiratory and Circulatory Systems

Respiratory System

The respiratory system provides the oxygen necessary for the body to metabolize fuel into the energies that are necessary for life. The word *pulmonary* refers to the lungs themselves, while the word *respiratory* refers to the structures that affect gas exchange (in this case, it includes the upper and lower airway structures).

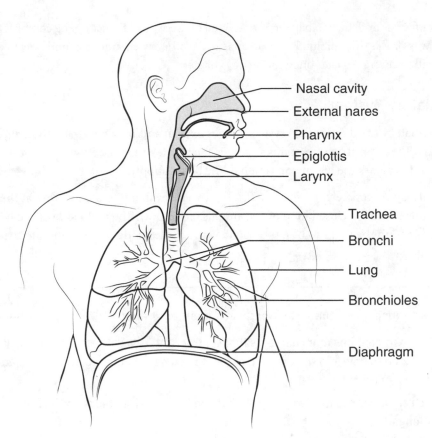

Labels:
- Nasal cavity
- External nares
- Pharynx
- Epiglottis
- Larynx
- Trachea
- Bronchi
- Lung
- Bronchioles
- Diaphragm

Figure 3.7 *Respiratory System*

The passage of air takes the path as follows:

- Air enters the nose through the **nasopharynx and nares** and the space behind the mouth called the **oropharynx**. Pharynx means space.

- At the inferior portion of the pharynx is the **epiglottis**, a leaflike valve that closes over the trachea during swallowing to prevent food and liquid from entering it.

- The **trachea** (windpipe) is the tube that connects the pharynx to the **bronchi**, which are the two tubes that lead into the lungs. The bronchi are surrounded by bands of muscle that help constrict or dilate the tubes to allow airflow in or out. Where the bronchi splits into the left and right side is called the **carina**. Further branches off the bronchi are called **bronchioles**.

- Vocal cords are located in the **larynx** (voice box). When expiratory air passes through this area, sound is made.

- The **diaphragm** and **intercostal muscles** contract and relax in order to pull air into the lungs.
  - **Negative pressure** is created when the diaphragm moves downward and allows the lungs to expand, which pulls in oxygen-rich air.
  - **Positive pressure** is created when the diaphragm relaxes and allows the lungs to contract, which forces carbon dioxide out.

- Oxygen and carbon dioxide move through the alveoli (grape-like sacs at the end of the bronchioles) through the permeable walls of the capillaries. This is called **gas exchange**.

In order for gas exchange to happen properly, all of these pieces must not be compromised in any way or else dysfunction begins to appear. Respiratory emergencies and how to assess them will be discussed later on in the airway chapter.

Circulatory System

The circulatory (cardiovascular) system carries oxygen and nutrients to all the cells of the body. The main structure of this system is the heart, which functions as a two-stage pump and provides the life-giving action of the blood supply.

The heart, approximately the size of a fist, has two sides that operate together at the same time, making a closed loop of continuous blood flow. The **right side** of the heart pumps blood to the lungs to be oxygenated, while the **left side** pumps blood to the rest of the body.

The heart pumps 5–6 quarts of blood each minute, or about 2,000 gallons per day.

- The heart contains four chambers that contract and relax at separate times, allowing blood to flow into the organ in order to become oxygenated and recirculated to the rest of the body.
- Each chamber has its own pathway that sends or receives blood to the body or lungs.

Path of Blood Flow

Questions about blood flow are some of the most commonly asked questions in class and on the NREMT exam. It is helpful to draw the pathway described below to help you memorize the route of blood.

1. Oxygen-poor blood enters the right atrium through both the superior and inferior vena cava.
2. As the atrium contracts, blood then flows downward through the open tricuspid valve, which empties into the right ventricle.
3. The right ventricle then contracts and pushes the blood through the pulmonic valve, which leads to the pulmonary arteries.
4. The pulmonary arteries allow the blood to enter into either the left or right lung, where gas exchange takes place at the capillary level of the alveoli.
5. Oxygen-rich blood is now returned through the pulmonary veins, which enter into the left atrium.
6. The left atrium contracts and squeezes blood downward through the open mitral valve, which empties into the left ventricle.
7. The left ventricle will then contract and send blood upward through the aortic valve into the aorta.
8. The aorta will then deliver blood to the rest of the body.

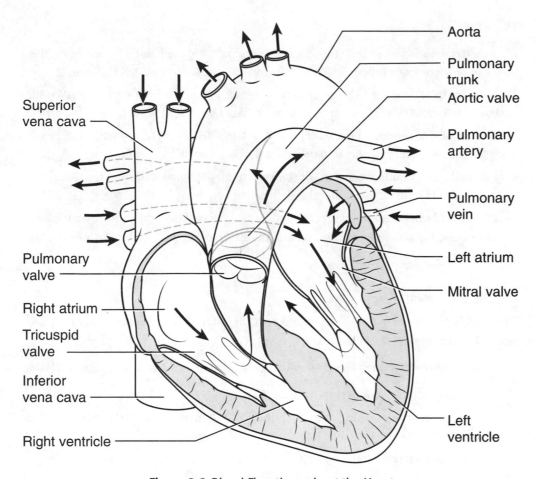

Figure 3.8 *Blood Flow throughout the Heart*

Electrical Pathway of the Heart

In order for the heart to pump blood correctly throughout the body, cardiac (myocardial) cells have specialized properties that allow electrical impulses to be generated and sent throughout the tissue in order to mechanically function. These properties are as follows:

- **Automaticity**: cell's ability to spontaneously generate an electrical impulse
- **Excitability**: cell's ability to respond to an electrical impulse
- **Conductivity**: cell's ability to transmit the electrical impulse to another cardiac cell
- **Contractility**: cell's ability of muscle to contract after an electrical impulse is received
- **Rhythmicity**: cell's ability to send electrical impulses in a regularly and evenly paced manner
- **Refractoriness**: cell's inability to respond to another electrical impulse

In order for these abilities to work properly, they need to be generated and filtered through an electrical pathway to all sections of the heart.

The pathway is as follows:

1. **Sinoatrial node (SA node)** (the "primary pacemaker of the heart") is located on the superior right side of the heart in the atrium. This causes a contraction motion.

2. **Atrioventricular node (AV node)**: signal is passed from the SA node to the AV node, which is located in the inferior portion of the right atrium, close to the right ventricle.

3. **Bundle of His**: located in the septal wall that separates the right and left ventricles. It splits the electrical pathway into two sides for each ventricle.

4. **Left and right bundle branches**: the two electrical pathways that stem from the bundle of His. They innervate either the right or left ventricle.

5. **Purkinje fibers** (small fibers) are located in the walls of the right and left ventricles. They cause the ventricles to contract and pump the blood into either the lungs or the rest of the body.

Vessels of the Heart

The heart has a system of both arteries and veins in order to create a loop of continuous blood flow throughout the body.

Arteries are vessels that carry blood **away from the heart**. The major arteries are as follows:

- **Coronary arteries**: connect to the heart itself
- **Aorta**: main artery coming out of the heart, which then bends 180 degrees into the trunk and divides at the navel into the two iliac arteries
- **Pulmonary artery**: carries blood from the right ventricle to the lungs
- **Carotid arteries**: supply blood to the brain
- **Femoral arteries**: supply blood to the lower extremities
- **Brachial arteries**: supply the upper arms and are used to listen for blood pressure, the pressure being generated by the pumping action of the heart
- **Radial arteries**: provide the lower arms and hands with blood

Veins are vessels that carry blood **to the heart**. The major veins are as follows:

- **Pulmonary vein**: carries oxygenated blood from the heart to the lungs
- **Superior vena cava**: carries blood from the head and upper extremities back to the heart
- **Inferior vena cava**: carries blood from the trunk and lower extremities to the heart

Sizing of Vessels

Vessels have different sizes throughout the body. From largest to smallest, sizing follows this pattern:

Arteries → arterioles → capillaries

Veins → venules → capillaries

Whether artery or vein, the smallest level is the **capillaries**. Found throughout the body, capillaries allow oxygen to pass into the adjacent cells and permit carbon dioxide (the waste by-product of the metabolic process) to pass from the cells into the blood.

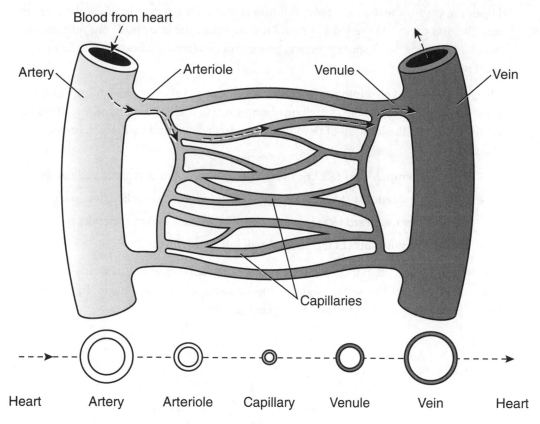

Figure 3.9 *Vessel Sizes*

Blood Components

Blood is made up of different cell types, each of which has a unique function in the body.

- **Red blood cells (RBCs)** carry oxygen, nutrients, and waste by-products.
- **White blood cells (WBCs)** (only 1% of the blood) are part of the body's defense mechanism against disease; they protect the body against illness and infection.
- **Platelets** allow blood to clot and thus stop leakage if a vessel has been damaged.
- **Plasma** (the clear fluid component of the blood, which contains all the cells mentioned above) helps to deliver nutrients to various organs and to remove waste products from the body.

Gastrointestinal and Genitourinary Systems

Gastrointestinal System

The gastrointestinal (GI) system—the body's fuel-processing plant—is comprised of the hollow organs in the trunk and abdomen.

Digestion begins the moment food or liquid (sometimes referred to as a bolus) enters into the oral cavity. As the food or liquid moves along, the body pulls out nutrients or water as it sees fit, with waste products being expelled from the body in the form of fecal matter.

The abdomen is divided into four quadrants, with the navel as its focal point. The EMT must know which organs lie in each quadrant, since in the event of blunt-force trauma to the abdomen, the location of rigidity and tenderness will indicate which organ is damaged.

- **Right upper quadrant (RUQ):** liver, right kidney, colon, pancreas, gallbladder
- **Left upper quadrant (LUQ):** liver, spleen, left kidney, stomach, colon, pancreas
- **Right lower quadrant (RLQ):** colon, small intestines, ureter, appendix
- **Left lower quadrant (LLQ):** colon, small intestines, ureter

The NREMT exam often includes questions about which organ lies in which quadrant, so do not skim over this section lightly. How to assess for various injuries in this area will be discussed in chapter 7, Trauma Emergencies.

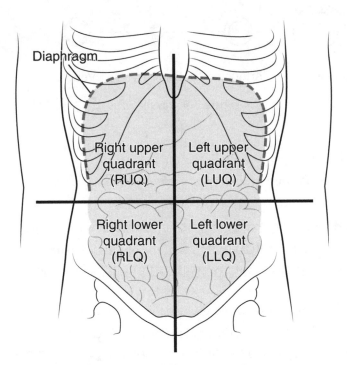

Figure 3.10 *Abdominal Quadrants*

Genitourinary System

The genitourinary (GU), or urogenital, system comprises the reproductive and urinary organs. Both male and female genitourinary systems have similar organs, with certain exceptions.

Urinary Organs

Whether the anatomy is male or female, the urinary portion of the system includes:

- **Kidneys** (two): responsible for filtering blood and producing urine
- **Ureters** (two): stem off from the kidney, allowing urine to pass through and flow into the bladder
- **Bladder**: has expansive properties; holds urine until it sends a signal through the nervous system to release
- **Urethra**: tube that carries urine from the bladder to the outside of the body; female urinary systems tend to have shorter urethras than male urinary systems

Only male urinary systems have a prostate gland, which surrounds the urethra. The gland's function is to secrete seminal fluid, needed for reproduction.

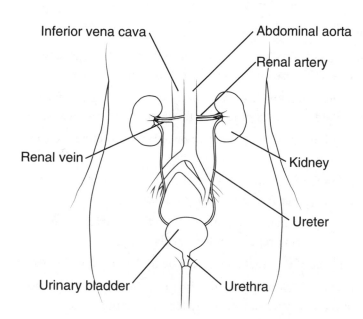

The female anatomy is the same as the male system, with the exception of the prostate gland and penis.

Figure 3.11 *Male Urinary System*

Reproductive Organs

Both male and female patients have reproductive organs that are very different from each other but have the same common purpose: to produce offspring in the form of an eventual fetus and subsequent child. Both male and female reproductive systems have organs that are located inside and outside of the body.

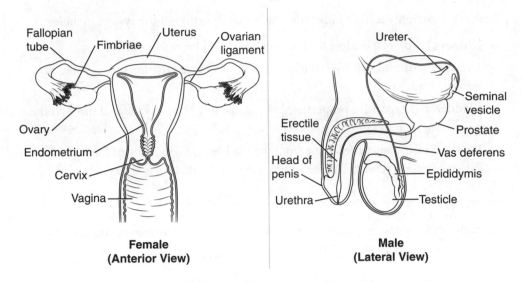

Figure 3.12 *Reproductive Organs*

Male Reproductive Organs

- **Testicles** (two of them, testes): responsible for creating and storing sperm cells; also part of the endocrine system because they produce the hormone testosterone

- **Prostate gland**: secretes fluid that nourishes and protects sperm; during ejaculation, the prostate squeezes this fluid into the urethra, and it's expelled with sperm as semen

- **Seminal vesicles**: along with the prostate gland, responsible for secreting most of the fluid that makes up semen

- **Epididymis**: tube located in the scrotum that is attached to the testicles; responsible for the transport and storing of sperm cells that are produced

- **Vas deferens**: tube that transports mature sperm to the urethra; carries urine or sperm to the outside of the body in preparation for ejaculation

- **Scrotum**: loose pouch-like sac of skin that hangs both behind and below the penis
  - Holds the testes and acts as a "climate control system," bringing the testes closer to the body for warmth and away from the body for cooling properties
  - Houses many nerves and blood vessels

- **Penis**: functional unit of reproduction in the male reproductive system. Cylindrical in shape, it is very vascular and made of spongy tissue that can become hard or soft depending on blood flow to the area. When the penis is erect, the flow of urine is blocked from the urethra, allowing only semen to be ejaculated at orgasm.

Hormones produced during the male reproductive cycle are as follows:

- **Follicle-stimulating hormone** (FSH) stimulates the production of sperm.

- **Luteinizing hormone** stimulates the production of testosterone.

- **Testosterone** is responsible for the development of male characteristics, e.g., muscle mass, body hair, sex drive.

Female Reproductive Organs

- **Labia majora and minora**: flaps of skin located on the outside of the vagina that protect the external organs
  - Minora (interior-facing): surrounds the opening of the vaginal canal and urethra
  - Majora (exterior-facing): as puberty progresses, will be covered with hair and will contain sweat and oil-producing glands
- **Clitoris**: where the labia minora meet is called the clitoris, which is a small, sensitive protrusion. It houses many nerves and can become erect tissue just like the penis.
- **Vagina**: a hollow canal that joins the cervix (the lower part of uterus) to the outside of the body. It also is known as the birth canal.
- **Uterus (womb)**: a hollow, pear-shaped organ consisting of vascular tissue that sheds in one of two ways:
  - Monthly (in the case of non-fertilization)
  - If fertilized, tissue does not shed and the corpus (main part of the uterus) expands, which then holds and helps develop the fetus
- **Ovaries** (two of them): small, oval-shaped glands located on either side of the uterus; responsible for producing eggs and hormones. When an egg is released, **fimbriae**, finger-like extensions, help push the egg from the ovary into the fallopian tube.
- **Fallopian tubes**: narrow tubes attached to the upper part of the uterus, which serve as passageways for the ova (egg cells) to travel from the ovaries to the uterus. If fertilization by sperm happens while the egg is still located in the fallopian tube, a dangerous condition called an ectopic pregnancy can occur.

Hormones produced during the female reproductive cycle are as follows:

- **Follicle-stimulating hormone**: as in male reproductive systems, but here it is responsible for production of egg growth in preparation for release from the ovary.
- **Luteinizing hormone**: as in male reproductive systems, but for female systems it triggers ovulation and development of the corpus luteum portion of the egg.
- **Estrogen**: as testosterone functions in male reproductive systems, estrogen regulates the menstrual cycle as well as helps develop female characteristics.
- **Progesterone**: secreted to prevent uterine contractions that may disturb the growing embryo; also prepares the breasts for lactation for feeding infants.

Nervous and Endocrine Systems

Nervous System

The nervous system is the central communication system for how the human body operates. Think of it as the "master computer." It is responsible for both voluntary and involuntary actions.

- **Neurons** are the building blocks of the brain. The neuron is the basic working unit of the brain, a specialized cell designed to transmit information to other nerve cells, muscle cells, or gland cells.

- **Dendrites** extend from the neuron cell body and receive messages from other neurons.
- **Synapses** are the contact points where one neuron communicates with another.
- A **nerve** is an enclosed, cable-like bundle of axons (the projections of neurons).

Follow the layout of the flowchart below in order to understand how the nervous system is broken down and how the parts of the nervous system relate to one another and cause various actions to occur.

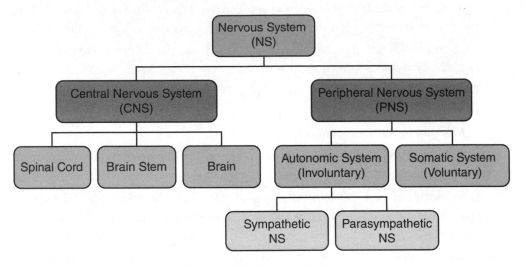

Figure 3.13 *Nervous System*

Central Nervous System

The first component is the **central nervous system (CNS)** consisting of the:

- **Brain**—this organ generates all the commands necessary for life such as breathing or the pumping of the heart.
- **Spinal cord**—this long cord is connected to the brain and has hundreds of nerves that innervate various organs and tissues. It is responsible for passing all signals from the brain to its target tissues.
- **Brain stem**—this is the bottom part of the brain and connects to the spinal cord. It controls the flow of messages sent from the brain to the rest of the body. It is responsible for regulation of cardiac and respiratory function, consciousness, and the sleep cycle.

Peripheral Nervous System

The second component is the peripheral nervous system (PNS), which is broken down into two systems, the **autonomic** and the **somatic nervous systems**.

The main function of the PNS is to connect the CNS to the limbs and organs, serving as an information highway between the brain, spinal cord, and the rest of the body. It includes 12 pairs of cranial nerves and 31 pairs of spinal nerves.

The autonomic nervous system is the part of the nervous system that controls and regulates the internal organs without any conscious recognition or effort, e.g., it functions involuntary and reflexively. It has two parts:

- **Sympathetic nervous system**: responsible for the "fight or flight" response, which prepares the body to expend energy and deal with potential threats in the environment
  - Will raise the heart rate, increase breathing rate, increase blood flow to muscles
  - Will activate sweat secretion
  - Will dilate the pupils
- **Parasympathetic system**: helps to maintain normal body functions and conserve physical resources
  - Will lower the heart rate, slow down breathing rate, decrease blood flow to muscles
  - Will constrict the pupils

Picture this example: You are taking a walk in the woods and come across a bear who starts to walk toward you. Your sympathetic nervous system will kick in and start to prepare you to either fight the bear or run away fast. Once the bear is gone and you are safe, your parasympathetic nervous system will allow you to calm down and come back to your normal resting state.

In other words, the parasympathetic nervous system "undoes" the work of the sympathetic division after a stressful event. It is responsible for the body's rest and digestion response when the body is relaxed, resting, or feeding.

The somatic system is responsible for carrying sensory and motor information to and from the central nervous system via two main types of neurons:

- Sensory neurons (or afferent neurons)—these carry information from the nerves to the CNS.
- Motor neurons (or efferent neurons)—these carry information from the brain and spinal cord to muscle fibers throughout the body.

Picture this example: You touch a hot stove burner with your bare hand. Your sensory neurons register "that's hot!" and send that message to your brain, which then sends the order back through motor neurons to snatch your hand away from the burner in order to stop the burning process.

Endocrine System

The endocrine system is made up of various glands that provide the body with the chemicals necessary for all bodily functions, such as insulin, adrenaline, and gender-specific hormones.

Table 3.2 *Endocrine Glands*

Gland Name	Location	Function
Pituitary (master gland)	Between the hypothalamus and the pineal gland, inside of the brain	Secretes hormones to control the other glands
Hypothalamus	Below the thalamus (a part of the brain that relays sensory information) and above the pituitary gland and brain stem	Secretes and metabolizes neuro-hormones, which either stimulate or inhibit the pituitary gland
Pineal	Deep in the center of the brain, in between the two halves of the brain	Secretes melatonin, which helps maintain circadian (sleep cycle) rhythm and regulate reproductive hormones
Thymus	Upper anterior part of your chest—directly behind the sternum and between the lungs	Stimulates development of T-cells, a specific type of white blood cell that is a major component of the immune system
Thyroid	Anterior neck	Controls metabolism
Parathyroid	Posterior to thyroid	Produces parathyroid hormone (PTH) for the metabolism of calcium and phosphorus in the bones
Adrenal	Sitting on top of (superior) to each kidney	Produces the chemicals adrenaline and norepinephrine, which are used by the nervous system and muscles to control energy and response to stimuli
Gonad (ovaries or testes)	Ovaries (located internally) are attached to the fallopian tubes; testes are located in the scrotum	Produces sex hormones
Pancreas (and islets of Langerhans)	Both in the upper left and right quadrant, posterior to the stomach	Produces insulin, which allows the body to metabolize sugar

Integumentary System

The integumentary system, more commonly known as skin, is the largest organ of the body. It is composed of three layers:

- **Epidermis**: outermost location and is most exposed of the layers
- **Dermis**: deeper layer containing sweat and sebaceous (oil-producing) glands, hair follicles, capillaries, and nerve endings
- **Subcutaneous/hypodermis**: below the dermis and contains fatty tissue

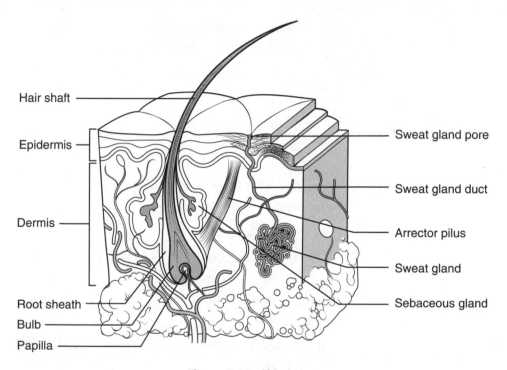

Hair shaft
Epidermis
Dermis
Root sheath
Bulb
Papilla

Sweat gland pore
Sweat gland duct
Arrector pilus
Sweat gland
Sebaceous gland

Figure 3.14 *Skin Layers*

The functions of the skin are as follows:

- Serves as the outer layer of the body and holds everything in place
- Serves to protect the entire body from the environment and outside organisms
- Via its sensory functions, provides the central nervous system with most of the required data for the brain to function appropriately and help the autonomic nervous system to properly regulate the body's temperature (crucial to cellular metabolism)

Practice Set

1. The patella is located in which anatomical plane?

   A. Inferior/posterior

   B. Inferior/anterior

   C. Superior/posterior

   D. Superior/anterior

2. The direction away from the midline in anatomical position is

   A. distal.

   B. medial.

   C. lateral.

   D. proximal.

3. Another name for the mandible is the

   A. cheekbone.

   B. jawbone.

   C. nose.

   D. eye socket.

4. _____ connect bones to bones.

   A. Tendons

   B. Smooth muscle

   C. Skeletal muscle

   D. Ligaments

5. How many vertebrae are located in the thoracic section of the spine?

   A. 6

   B. 12

   C. 18

   D. 19

6. In respiratory inspiration, air passes through the pharynx into the

   A. nasopharynx.

   B. oropharynx.

   C. trachea.

   D. esophagus.

7. What is the name of a cardiac cell's ability to generate its own electrical impulse?

   A. Automaticity

   B. Elasticity

   C. Excitability

   D. Rhythmicity

8. Which of the following is NOT a part of the respiratory system?

   A. Aorta

   B. Nasopharynx

   C. Trachea

   D. Alveoli

9. At which age do fontanelles typically close in the skull?

   A. 6 months

   B. 12 months

   C. 24 months

   D. 18 months

10. Which type of muscle would be responsible for the digestion of food in the gastrointestinal system?

    A. Skeletal

    B. Smooth

    C. Cardiac

    D. Pulmonary

11. Which of the following accurately describes the function of the peripheral nervous system?

    A. Transmits information from the central nervous system to the limbs and organs

    B. Processes information received from the sensory organs and orchestrates the appropriate action

    C. Regulates the excretion of epinephrine

    D. Responsible for the "fight or flight" response

12. Which organ is responsible for housing sensory nerves, regulating body temperature, and protecting the body's organs from the environment?

    A. Kidney

    B. Brain

    C. Skin

    D. Liver

13. The main artery coming from the left ventricle is called the

    A. aorta.

    B. pulmonary artery.

    C. inferior vena cava.

    D. superior vena cava.

14. Deoxygenated blood enters which heart chamber from the vena cava?

    A. Right atrium

    B. Left atrium

    C. Right ventricle

    D. Left ventricle

15. The focal electrical site that causes the ventricles to contract is called the

    A. sinoatrial node.

    B. atrioventricular node.

    C. Purkinje node.

    D. node of His.

16. What are the main functional units of the brain called?

    A. Neurons

    B. Nerves

    C. Synapses

    D. Dendrites

17. Which gland is most affected by diabetes?

    A. Adrenal

    B. Pituitary

    C. Pancreas

    D. Thyroid

18. Your ambulance responds to a motor vehicle accident. When you arrive, you find a male patient who was unrestrained and struck the dash. The upper left abdominal quadrant is tender and slightly rigid. You note a large bruise also in the upper left quadrant. The other abdominal quadrants are soft with no tenderness or rigidity. What injury should you suspect?

    A. Ruptured appendix

    B. Liver laceration

    C. Perforated bladder

    D. Spleen laceration

19. What plane divides the body into the left and right side?

    A. Sagittal

    B. Frontal

    C. Transverse

    D. Midaxillary

20. The phalanges are _____ to the elbow.

    A. proximal

    B. superior

    C. lateral

    D. distal

21. Which hormone is responsible for stimulating sperm production in males and egg growth in females?

    A. Follicle-stimulating hormone

    B. Luteinizing hormone

    C. Epinephrine

    D. Growth hormone

22. Which layer of the skin is most susceptible to superficial damage such as an abrasion or burn?

    A. Hypodermis

    B. Subcutaneous

    C. Dermis

    D. Epidermis

23. You are dispatched to a call for a broken hip of a 77-year-old female. Upon arrival at her home, you find the patient laying on the ground in her bedroom in the supine position. You notice that her right leg is at a strange angle and appears to be turning inward. This injury would be a result of what type of movement?

    A. Pronation

    B. Rotation

    C. Supination

    D. Abduction

24. During an assessment, when you ask for the patient to point the toes toward the ground, you are asking for which movement and in which plane?

    A. Extension; sagittal

    B. Dorsiflexion; transverse

    C. Extension; frontal

    D. Plantar flexion; sagittal

25. You are called to the fifth floor of an apartment building for an unknown-type medical call. Upon arrival, you find a male patient in the tripod position and in obvious respiratory distress. After your partner places oxygen on him at your request, you begin to listen to lung sounds. You hear wheezing bilaterally, which means which lung structures are MOST likely being affected the greatest?

    A. Alveoli

    B. Carina

    C. Capillaries

    D. Bronchi

26. In order from smallest to largest, what are the sizes of veins?

    A. Capillaries, veins, venules

    B. Venules, capillaries, veins

    C. Veins, capillaries, venules

    D. Capillaries, venules, veins

Answers and Explanations

1. B

This question tests your knowledge of the anatomical planes and anatomical names. Once you have determined that the patella is the kneecap, you then can place it on the front (anterior) side of the leg, which is inferior to the horizontal midline of the body.

2. C

Distal does mean away from, but since the midline is the point in question, the correct answer is lateral. *Medial* means toward the midline and *proximal* means next to. It is helpful to remember the pairs, such as lateral/medial, superior/inferior, etc., rather than try to memorize them individually.

3. B

The cheekbone is the zygomatic bone. The nose is not a bone, but consists of cartilage, and the eye socket is the orbit. A good way to learn anatomy is to purchase an anatomy coloring book.

4. D

Ligaments connect bones to other bones in order to form joints. Tendons connect muscles to bones. The other two muscles exist in the body but have specific functions not related to connecting bones together.

5. B

The correct answer is 12. This is a common question on the NREMT exam.

6. C

The nasopharynx and oropharynx are parts of the pharynx located posterior to the nose and mouth, respectively. Oxygenated air then enters the trachea through the vocal cords past the epiglottis. The epiglottis closes over the esophagus to prevent air from entering the gastrointestinal system.

7. A

The correct answer is automaticity. Elasticity is not a term associated with cardiac cells. Excitability is the ability to respond to an electrical impulse. Finally, rhythmicity may seem like a good answer, but it has to do with sending the pulses generated in an evenly spaced manner.

8. A

The correct answer is aorta, which is part of the heart.

9. D

Remember that fontanelles are specialized to pediatric patients. They are where the sutures of the skull have not fully stitched themselves together yet to form the overall hard cranial cap. The correct answer is 18 months.

10. B

The digestive process works without our having to consciously will it to happen. (D) is not a muscle, so this rules out this answer—*pulmonary* is another word used to describe the respiratory system. We know that cardiac means "heart," so we're left with skeletal or smooth muscle. Skeletal muscles are used to move our bones around, while smooth muscle is used to move fluids (or broken-down food) around our body through rhythmic contractions and relaxation.

11. A

The peripheral nervous system is responsible for transmitting information from the central nervous system to the muscles and various organs of the body. The other definitions describe the functions of the autonomic nervous system.

12. C

The skin is the largest organ in the body and is responsible for housing sensory nerves, regulating body temperature, and protecting organs from the environment. None of the other answers are organs that perform these functions.

13. A

Both the superior and inferior vena cava are considered two of the greater-sized veins in the body, so while they do help bring blood to the heart, they are neither an artery nor do they attach to the left ventricle. This leaves you with (A) or (B). The correct answer is the main artery supplying the body with oxygenated blood, the aorta.

14. A

The answer is the right atrium. Blood always enters into the atrium first, on either side depending on the pathway of flow the blood is currently at. The ventricles are the bottom two chambers of the heart and are responsible for the strong contractions to push the blood to either the body (left side) or the lungs (right side).

15. B

Sinoatrial contains the word *atrial,* which refers to the atrium, or upper part of the heart, so we can rule that one out. There is no such thing as the Purkinje node or node of His; however, after the electrical command passes through the atrioventricular node, it then passes through the bundle of His into the Purkinje fibers. The only answer that contains the root *ventricle* is atrioventricular, so that is likely the correct answer.

16. A

We can rule out (B) as while nerves are parts of the nervous system in general, they are not specifically located in the brain itself. (D) is a part of a neuron, but (A), the entire neuron itself, is the functional unit of the brain. (C) is the connection point where two or more neurons "speak" to one another.

17. C

With diabetes, the body ceases to produce the hormone insulin, and that affects the body's ability to metabolize sugar into energy. It also affects the islets of Langerhans, which are located within the pancreas. The adrenal gland produces epinephrine (adrenaline) and norepinephrine, which affect the nervous system; the pituitary gland secretes multiple hormones that control various glands and processes; and the thyroid helps regulate metabolism.

18. D

The spleen is located in the upper left quadrant, and there should be a high index of suspicion of damage to the spleen with any trauma to this abdominal quadrant. The liver is located mostly in the upper right quadrant. The bladder is located in the lower quadrants. The appendix is located in the lower right quadrant.

19. A

The frontal plane divides the body into anterior and posterior, and also contains the reference point of the midaxillary line. The transverse plane divides the body into superior and inferior portions. Refer back to the table in the anatomical directions and planes section to refresh your memory if you got this question wrong.

20. D

When speaking about limbs, we mainly use proximal and distal to describe structures in relation to one another. Proximal means "closer to" the trunk of the body while distal means "farther away from." Think of the word *distance* when trying to remember the difference between the two. Superior (B) refers to something above, which would be a good guess here, but is not appropriate for this particular question.

21. A

Your first thought may have been (D) since it contains the word *growth*. However, growth hormone is not specific to the reproductive system. Luteinizing hormone (B) is a reproductive hormone but is responsible for stimulation of testosterone or triggering of ovulation. Epinephrine (C) is a hormone but is not specific to the reproductive system. That leaves follicle-stimulating hormone (A), which is found in both male and female reproductive systems; it affects pubertal development and the function of ovaries and testes.

22. D

Both (A) and (B) are called the same layer of skin, depending on which anatomist or textbook you use. It is the deepest layer of the skin. The dermis is where most of the "parts" are, such as veins, arteries, nerves, sweat glands, etc. The key to this question is the word "superficial," which means "occurring at or near the surface," and that means that the epidermis, (D), would be the correct answer as it is the top layer of skin.

23. B

Abduction (D) is a movement made in the frontal plane and involves moving a body part toward or away from the midline. While this may seem like a good choice, you are looking for a rotational type of movement (B) as the hip uses a ball and socket joint in order to move properly. Both (A) and (C) also rotate, but around another bone to achieve their movements.

24. D

As the movement is happening with either the left or right foot, this puts us in the sagittal plane. So, any answer that does not include the sagittal plane can be ruled out. Both dorsiflexion and plantar flexion have to do with the foot in particular, so this leaves you with two choices, even if you are unsure of which plane. Putting these two strategies together, you get correct answer (D).

25. D

The bronchi are two tubes that have bands of muscle that constrict or dilate to allow air flow in or out of the lungs. In this case, this patient's bronchi are being constricted, which is creating a smaller space for air to pass and produces a wheezing sound. He needs a bronchodilator medication to relieve this. While the rest of the answer choices are located in the respiratory system, they are not the MOST affected as the question asks.

26. D

(D) is the correct answer. Please refer back to the circulatory system and sizing of vessels portion of this chapter to see a visual aid if you got this question wrong.

CHAPTER 4

Patient Assessment and Documentation

Topics Discussed

- Scene Size-Up Considerations
- Initial Patient Assessment Components
- Obtaining Baseline Vital Signs
- SAMPLE and OPQRST
- Performing a Focused History and Physical Exam: Medical and Trauma
- Detailed Physical Exam Components and Ongoing Patient Assessment
- Radio Communications and Documentation

It is just after midnight when your radio beeps and dispatch announces, "Rescue 1, respond to 123 Main Street, unknown-type medical call, no other information available." You pull on your examination gloves and respond with lights and sirens to the call.

An unknown-type medical call is a truly random event, and you can encounter something as simple as a splinter in a finger or as dangerous as an ongoing gun battle. Dispatchers are trained to try and get as much information as they can from a caller, but the information they are given may be fragmented or incomplete, especially if the call is coming from a third party.

Patient Assessment

Patient assessment is the most important part of your toolbox as an EMT. It's not enough to be able to only visually see symptoms or signs. You must know how to ask specific questions to determine the true issue a patient is suffering from.

It's like being a medical detective. From the moment you are dispatched to the moment you clear yourself from a call, assessment is not a one-time event. Let's review the different parts.

Scene Size-Up

Here are some guidelines for assessing the scene. This information may be critical to patient care or even a police investigation.

Assess for Hazards

As an EMT you must be able to ascertain to the best of your ability whether a scene is safe, and you always want to err on the side of caution. You see a person down and your first inclination is to run right over and render care, but even before you get out of the truck, you must scan the area and see if there are any hazards present that would endanger your safety or the safety of your crew.

These hazards may be people who present a danger, such as a person with a weapon; hazardous materials, such as toxic or dangerous chemicals; or environmental hazards, such as unstable ground, ice, or snow. If you determine a scene is unsafe, it must be made safe before entering.

Observe the Scene

Once the scene has been made safe, you should be observant of all that is around you. This observation will also assist you in determining whether this is a medical call or a trauma call, since that determination will be important in how you assess and treat your patient. Always do the following:

- When you approach a scene, you must act as a medical detective, looking for the clues which will allow you to treat this situation properly. If conscious and alert, the patient is usually the best source of information. If this is not the case, then bystanders become your next best source. Don't ignore the people standing around if you cannot ascertain from the victim what the problem is.

- The number of patients is also a concern that has to be dealt with immediately. The number of patients and the severity of injury or illness will help determine how many additional units will be needed at this event.

- If this is a medical call, then the nature of the illness must be determined as soon as you have established that the patient has an airway, is breathing, and has a pulse (ABC). If you determine that this is a trauma call, then you must next determine what the mechanism of injury is, or how this patient became injured. Again, ABCs must be checked first (see below).

Don't get tunnel vision when encountering a seriously injured patient. An open femur fracture is sure to get your attention, but if you treat it with a traction splint and forget to check for an open airway you may deliver a dead patient to the ED with a properly applied traction splint.

Injuries such as these are referred to as "distracting injuries." They may look bad, but they will cause you to miss other more important, life-threatening injuries.

Initial Patient Assessment

Remember Your ABCs

As you approach a patient, ideally from the feet, observe him or her to determine priority, age, gender, and overall appearance.

- Introduce yourself as an EMT and ask the patient his or her name.
- If the patient is conscious and responsive, that will tell you right away that the patient has an airway, is breathing, and has circulation (ABC).
- If the patient is unconscious, first check the airway, open it if necessary, ventilate if apneic, and ascertain whether there is a pulse.

Always treat life-threatening situations as you encounter them. If the patient has no pulse, commence CPR immediately.

Level of Consciousness

If the patient has no immediate life-threatening conditions, you must then determine what level of consciousness exists. This can be remembered by the acronym **AVPU**.

- Fully **A**lert (responds appropriately to a normal voice)
- Responsive to **V**erbal stimuli (responds only if spoken to in a loud voice)
- Responsive to **P**ainful stimuli (responds only to a vigorous rub of the sternum or something similar)
- **U**nconscious (does not respond to any of the above)

Bleeding Control

With ABCs taken care of and level of consciousness established, the EMT must next check for gross hemorrhage or major bleeding. If these are present, steps must be taken to control the bleeding. Specific techniques will be discussed in the trauma section.

Pulse Check

You should be familiar with the major anatomical points for palpating a pulse. These include the radius at the wrist, the brachia in the upper arm, the posterior tibial and dorsalis pedal in the feet, the carotid in the neck, and the femoral in the upper leg.

While the most common pulse point checked is either the radial or carotid pulse in adults and the brachial in pediatrics, knowing that you have options is useful if one of the more common points is not available for some reason such as trauma or inability to locate a palpable pulse.

Temperature

As you are assessing, feel the patient's forehead and exposed areas of skin on arms and legs, if appropriate, for temperature. Using the back of your hand is ideal for this.

The skin should be warm and dry. If it is hot to the touch, then the patient may be running a fever or have been exposed to high temperatures. If cold, then the patient may be hypothermic from cold exposure or have circulation impairment. Is the skin dry or moist? Dampness may be due to **diaphoresis**, or sweating, a symptom of many medical problems.

Transport Priority Decision

The initial assessment is performed primarily to indicate whether the patient should be transported immediately or if there is time to perform a more thorough assessment on scene and perform any applicable treatment protocols. A patient who presents as being in serious condition should be transported immediately, with any further assessment and/or intervention done en route to the emergency department.

In addition, the following are considered "load and go" patients based on the primary assessment:

- Unresponsive with no gag reflex
- Responsive but unable to follow commands
- Dyspnea (difficulty breathing)
- Hypoperfusion syndrome (shock)
- Childbirth with complications
- Chest pains with pallor and dyspnea
- Uncontrolled hemorrhaging
- Severe pain

Any of the above conditions would require a priority transport. Immobilize the patient if needed and transport to the nearest emergency department. Depending on the situation, you could also consider requesting an ALS intercept to initiate advanced protocols with less loss of time to the patient. (As the primary consideration is *time lost*, if you can get to the emergency department faster than it would take for ALS to arrive, then of course do that.)

If the situation is not a priority transport, then the EMT proceeds to the appropriate focused assessment and physical examination. This is sometimes called a "stay and play" situation, with the word play meaning certain treatments or focused assessments may be done on scene without the immediate danger of the patient degrading on scene.

Be aware that at any time the patient's condition may change, or the focused assessment may discover a condition that necessitates an immediate transport. If that happens, transport without delay.

Initially, the EMT should determine the chief complaint, which can be asked in various ways, but watch your tone and body language. Your goal is to make the patient feel comfortable about your intervention, but also to get all the vital information needed.

- **DO NOT ask**, "Why are we here?" standing over the patient, with hands on the hips.
- **DO ask**, "How can I help you? Can you explain what happened?" sitting/squatting at the patient's eye level, with kindness in your voice.

A helpful mnemonic that is taught to all EMS professionals is the SAMPLE set of questions. This is a concise way to get a lot of information about the patient and the reason why 911 was called for assistance.

Questions you ask should not be simply a "checklist" of facts. You need to understand the *story* of what happened. Piece together the different details you learn to get a larger picture so that you can determine the proper course of treatment.

If the patient is unconscious or otherwise unable to respond, then bystanders and/or family members are the best resource for this assessment.

Once the immediate problem is stated, ask six questions to get a better picture (the **SAMPLE** history). Let's assume your patient is a female who says she has abdominal pain.

- Signs and symptoms
  - **Is it like anything you've had before?**
  - **Can you point to exactly where it hurts? Does anything make the pain better or worse?**
  - The focus of your questions should be on the multiple causes for female abdominal pain, e.g., a gastrointestinal, vascular, or gynecologic condition. If the patient says that she developed a sharp pain in her right lower quadrant an hour ago, and she is holding her hand on the right lower abdomen just superior to the right leg, you may want to suspect appendicitis. Do not assume anything, however, and ask the remainder of the questions.
- Allergies
  - **Do you have any allergies?**
  - This is pretty straightforward. Most people are willing to share this information.
- Medications
  - **Are you on any medications?**
  - This starts to get confidential. Some patients will provide a negative answer and then, in the privacy of the emergency department, tell the nurse the truth. This is especially true for medications for sexually transmitted diseases, HIV, hepatitis, or erectile dysfunction.

- Also keep in mind any over the counter (OTC) medications such as pills, powders, tinctures, homemade or homeopathic medications. Sometimes these may be causing a reaction for someone, but because they are not prescribed by a medical doctor, patients may not think of them as "medications."

- Pertinent history

  - **Are you being treated for any medical conditions?**

  - If the patient with abdominal pain now says that she has a history of ulcerative colitis, you may need to rethink your assumption about appendicitis. Again, certain conditions may cause patients to not tell you the truth. Be alert for signs of lying, such as the inability to maintain eye contact or a sudden change in demeanor.

  - If you think that the patient is telling a serious lie, be sure to share your suspicions with the triage nurse at the emergency department. The goal is not to catch someone in a lie, but rather to ensure that a true clinical picture emerges for the physician who will treat your patient.

  - Make sure to keep your patient focused on major and most recent medical history, especially if they are elderly or have psychological issues that may lead to an extensive history.

- Last oral intake

  - **When and what did you last eat?**

  - If the patient says that she ate "two large orders of super hot chicken wings a few hours ago," you might want to consider that her gastric pain may be caused by indigestion.

- Events leading to this episode

  - **What happened just prior to the pain starting?**

  - This may give you a clue to the current condition. A female experiencing abdominal pain could have multiple causes—from medical to traumatic reasons. Gaining a clear picture in the patient's own words could help clarify why she may be experiencing the pain. Ask about her menstrual cycle, possible pregnancy status, and any recent physical trauma, which can help to narrow down the possibilities.

Baseline Vital Signs

- **Level of consciousness** is determined by asking the patient questions and recording whether the answers are appropriate.

  - These questions should relate to person, place, time, and event.

  - Sample questions include, "What is your name?" "Do you know where you are?" "Do you know what day it is?" and "Do you know what happened to bring you to this situation?"

  - If the answers to the questions are satisfactory, then the patient is said to be **alert and oriented times 4.**

  - If the answers to the questions are unsatisfactory, i.e., if the patient is unable to state what happened, then the notation would be **alert and oriented times 3, with confusion as to present event.**

- **Pulse rate** in an adult patient is usually measured by finding the pulse at the point where the radial artery crosses the wrist bone.
  - You may count the number of beats for 15 seconds, multiplying by 4.
  - You may also count for 30 seconds and multiply by 2.
  - If the pulse is irregular, count the pulse for a full minute and make a notation that it is irregular.
- **Respiratory rate** is calculated by watching the rise and fall of the patient's chest wall for 15 seconds, and then multiplying by 4.
  - If the rate is irregular, take the measurement for a full minute.
  - If the breathing is shallow, deep, or labored, or if you can hear noises as the patient breathes (e.g., wheezing, snoring sounds, or high pitched whistling sounds), that indicates a potentially serious medical problem.
  - An option is to act as if you are taking a radial pulse and fold their arm at the elbow, placing it against their chest. You can then feel the chest rise and fall and count respirations without having to stare at the person, who may become self-conscious and breathe at a different pace or pattern.
- **Blood pressure** is measured by placing a blood pressure cuff (sphygmomanometer) on the upper arm and listening with a stethoscope over the brachial artery inside of the elbow. The cuff is inflated to 200 mm of mercury, and then the pressure is slowly released.
  - The point at which the pulse sound begins to be heard is the systolic blood pressure, or the pressure in the arteries as the ventricles in the heart contract and push blood into the system.
  - As the pressure in the cuff continues to drop, the sound grows louder and then begins to diminish.
  - When the sound cannot be heard any longer, diastolic pressure, or the pressure in the arteries while the ventricles are at rest, is taken.
- In documenting **skin condition**, note the **skin color**, temperature, and condition. The color of the skin indicates many things and is often the most useful diagnostic tool available to the EMT.
  - Is the patient pale, cyanotic (bluish), flushed (red), or jaundiced (yellow)?
    - In patients with little or no pigmentation, changes in skin color may be more easily observed due to the lack of melanin in the skin.
    - In patients with deeply pigmented skin, changes in skin color may be apparent only in certain areas, such as the fingernail beds, the lips, the mucous membranes in the mouth, the underside of the arm/hand, and the conjunctiva of the eye.
    - It can also be helpful to ask patients themselves (or someone who knows them) if their color appears different than usual.
  - Is the patient's skin cool, normal temperature, or warm to the touch?
  - Is the skin dry, or is the patient sweating (diaphoretic)?

- **Capillary refill** is a measure of how the patient is perfusing, i.e., how well oxygen is being transferred from the red blood cells to the tissues.
  - Measured by depressing the nail bed and noting how many seconds elapse before the color returns.
  - Normal return of color should be 2 seconds or less; longer than that and it is considered delayed.
- **Pupils** often reveal information about the condition of the patient's nervous system. Shine a pocket flashlight into each eye and note the following:
  - Do the pupils contract and then dilate as you move the light out of the pupil?
  - Are the pupils of equal size and shape?
  - Can the patient follow the moving light from side to side with the eyes?

Documenting the pupils can be done in various ways:

- **PERL**: Pupils Equal Reactive to Light
- **PERRL**: Pupils Equal, Round, and Reactive to Light
- **PERLA**: Pupils Equal, Round, Reactive to Light, and Accommodating

Focused History and Physical Exam: Medical

Regardless of whether you have decided to prioritize transport or not, the next step is to conduct a focused history and physical exam of the patient.

Vital Signs

If you have not already taken a baseline set of vitals, this is the time to do so. A blood glucose level (BGL) reading may also be taken at this time if permitted by local protocol, especially in cases of altered consciousness.

Patient Complaints

Next is the assessment of the patient's complaints and signs and symptoms. Naturally, these questions cannot be answered if the patient is unresponsive, unless a witness/family member can assist.

The acronym OPQRST is helpful for remembering what to ask about the condition that has brought EMS to this patient.

- **Onset**: when did the pain start?
- **Provocation**: is there anything the patient does that aggravates the problem?
- **Quality**: can the patient describe the pain?
- **Radiation**: does the pain move in any direction?
- **Severity**: how bad is the pain on a scale of 1 to 10 (worst)?
- **Time**: how long has the pain persisted, and is this the first time it is happening?

Let's say you respond to a patient with chest pain. Scene safety, universal precautions, and ABCs are all done, and the primary assessment gives you no indication for a need to expedite transport. Since your patient is conscious and alert, now is the time to ask these questions. They will help to facilitate a discussion about what the patient is experiencing.

TEST YOURSELF 4.1

Using the OPQRST questions, how would you label this patient's response for each letter?

"The pain started right after I finished exercising an hour ago. I was lifting weights, and all of a sudden I felt a sharp pain right here [points to left chest superior to his left nipple]. If I raise my left arm, it gets a lot worse, and it feels like a tearing sensation. The pain doesn't move. I would rate it about 6 on a scale of 1 to 10. I've never had anything like it before."

What do you think this patient is suffering from, given his answers for chest pain?

At this point, you should have a general clinical picture of what the condition is and be ready to conduct a thorough physical exam.

- It is not necessary to palpate the entire body of a patient; however, it is necessary to physically examine the area of complaint.
- Palpating with the fingertips is often revealing as to what the ultimate diagnosis will be. Does the area of complaint appear normal in relation to the surrounding body areas? When you feel it with your fingers, does it feel the same as the surrounding tissue or is it abnormally rigid?
- When you palpate, does the patient complain that the area you are touching is tender or painful? Pain that is increasing or decreasing is a sign of something wrong.

At the conclusion of the focused medical assessment, if the patient is unconscious, position the patient to protect the airway and transport the patient to the hospital emergency department. Remember that assessment is constant and repeated often, and you should be alert during the transport for changes in the patient's status and prepared to respond accordingly.

Focused Physical Exam: Trauma

The detailed physical exam (or the head-to-toe exam) enables the EMT to get a clearer picture of what is going on with the patient. In the past, the purpose of the exam was to identify and treat life-threatening conditions and stabilize the patient. Now, however, a more complete exam is used to reveal conditions that will be of help to the receiving physician so that a definitive diagnosis can be made and treatment can be started.

Each EMT will develop a personalized system for performing a complete physical assessment. The goal should always be a methodical and thorough checking of the entire external body.

Head-to-Toe Exam

The mnemonic **DCAP-BTLS** is used as each section of the body is closely examined both visually and by touch.

- **D**eformities; **C**ontusions; **A**brasions; **P**unctures/Penetrations
- **B**urns; **T**enderness; **L**acerations; **S**welling

A thorough exam includes the following, while checking for DCAP-BTLS at each section.

Table 4.1 *Detailed Physical Exam*

Body Section	Palpate/Check For	Possible Injury or Condition
Head	• Cranial plate instability • Fluids coming out of ears, nose, or mouth • Bruising behind the ears (Battle sign)	• Skull fracture • Internal cranial injury
Face	• Traumatic injury and bleeding • Pupil response, color, and foreign bodies	• Internal head structural injury • Internal head bleed • Concussion • Increased cranial pressure • Poisoning • Overdose
Nose and Mouth	• Fluids • Loose or broken teeth • Foreign odors	• Fluid buildup: saliva or blood • Lacerations from broken teeth • Airway obstruction from loose teeth or difficulty getting a good mask seal if needed • Odors (could indicate alcohol intoxication or ketones in diabetic emergencies)
Neck	• Jugular vein distension • Tracheal shift • Subcutaneous emphysema (bubbling sensation under the skin)	• Tension pneumothorax • Underlying air leakage from the respiratory system secondary to chest trauma or illness
Chest	• Rib tenderness, crepitus • Paradoxical motion (an area of the chest moves in the opposite direction of normal motion)	• Rib fracture • Flail segment ($\geq$2 ribs are broken in $\geq$2 places)

(Continued)

Table 4.1 *Detailed Physical Exam (Continued)*

Body Section	Palpate/Check For	Possible Injury or Condition
Abdomen	• Bounding or visible pulsation around the naval • If patient complains of pain, start palpating away from the pain first • Palpate all 4 quadrants, feeling for rigid or soft feeling	• Rigidity (could indicate intra-abdominal bleed) • Bounding or visual pulsation (could indicate an abdominal aortic aneurysm, which could be fatal if ruptured)
Pelvis/Genitalia	• Stability (pelvis): gently compress and press down on either hip • Bleeding or priapism (persistent erection in male genitalia)	• Hip fracture, including "open book" fracture (would cause a lot of blood to collect in pelvic cavity) • Priapism (could indicate spinal injury in males) • Internal or external bleeding on genitalia must be padded and controlled by pressure
Arms/Legs (extremities)	• Pulse and capillary refill in each extremity • Motor function: "Squeeze my hand" or "Wiggle your toes." • Sensation: "Can you feel this?" or "Which finger or toe am I touching?"	• Circulatory compromise if delayed capillary refill • Dislocated bones/joints • Impaired motor or sensory function could indicate spinal injury
Back/Posterior	• Injury to the spine/back • Must be done while log-rolling patient onto the backboard (not while patient is secured onto backboard)	• Spinal injury • DCAP-BTLS injuries

The final step in the detailed assessment is to retake vital signs and note especially any wide divergence from the initial vital signs taken during the focused assessment.

Scores

There are two methods used in EMS to score an assessment. Either one can help you to monitor changing conditions in the patient and to determine transport priority/destination. Since the patient's status can change at any time, you must be diligent in your reassessment to catch any developing issues.

Glasgow Coma Scale (GCS) assesses a patient's level of consciousness in both medical and traumatic injury. GCS calculation is made by assigning the following index numbers as appropriate. The range is 3–15 total points. A patient who is unconscious and unresponsive would receive a score of 3, while a patient who shows no deficiencies would receive a score of 15.

Table 4.2 *Calculating the Glasgow Coma Scale*

Type of Response Tested	Points Assigned
Eye Response	• Spontaneous (4) • To verbal stimuli (3) • To painful stimuli (2) • No response (eyes will not open) (1)
Verbal Response	• Oriented conversation (5) • Confused conversation (4) • Inappropriate conversation (3) • Incomprehensible conversation (2) • No response (1)
Motor Response	• Obeys commands (6) • Localizes pain (5) • Withdraws from pain (4) • Flexes extremities/decorticate position (3) • Extends extremities/decerebrate position (2) • No response (1)

Revised Trauma Score (RTS) is a numerical index based on the severity of injury and patient condition in a traumatic injury. RTS calculation takes into account the systolic blood pressure, respiratory rate, and the GCS score. The range is 1–12 total points.

Table 4.3 *Calculating the Revised Trauma Score (RTS)*

Measurement Taken	Points Assigned
Respiratory Rate	• 10–29 breaths per minute (4) • Greater than 29 breaths per minute (3) • 6–9 breaths per minute (2) • 1–5 breaths per minute (1)
Systolic Blood Pressure	• >89 mm (4) • 77–89 mm (3) • 50–75 mm (2) • 1–75 mm (1) • No pulse or no blood pressure (0)
GCS Score	• 13–15 (4) • 9–12 (3) • 6–8 (2) • 4–5 (1) • <4 (0)

TEST YOURSELF 4.2

Calculate the Revised Trauma Score for the following patient:

- Conscious: GCS score of 14
- Respiratory rate 20/min
- Blood pressure 80/60 mm Hg

Ongoing Reassessment

Once initial and focused assessments are complete, if the patient is still in the care of the EMT then the responsibility for the patient remains with that EMT. This is the portion of the call during which the patient's condition can change and not be noticed, often with tragic results. Apnea can occur without any struggle or outward sign, and should that happen the EMT must be ready to deal with this new medical problem. A patient who is stable one minute could conceivably, and often will, become unstable in the next.

As a general rule:

- Repeat vital signs every 5 minutes for unstable patients and every 10–15 minutes for stable patients. (These should be entered chronologically in the patient documentation care report.)
- Repeat the focused assessment anytime you detect a change in patient condition.
- Repeat the focused assessment if a downgrading trend is noticed, whether vital signs or mental status.

As new conditions occur, they must be treated as encountered, and the receiving facility must be notified immediately of the new information.

Documentation

In addition to the legal considerations, good documentation is also a prerequisite for good patient care. Depending on your service and location, *documentation* may be called various things. In this section, we will refer to documentation using different terms, but they are all referring to the same thing—information that is collected on a patient, what occurred during the call, and a document that is either in paper or digital format submitted to your service for billing purposes.

Prehospital Care Report

The documentation of an EMS encounter is called a prehospital care report (PCR), but is commonly referred to as a **run report** or just "chart." Many agencies have moved away from paper charting and now utilize electronic versions, also called EPCRs or ePCRs.

It is your responsibility to be familiar with the format of charting that your agency uses and be able to fill out a report on each and every patient you treat. The general rule of documentation is that if it's not written down, it didn't happen.

The bane of any job is paperwork, and EMS charts are no exception. Since you, as an EMT, are in a medical profession and the United States is the most litigious country in the world, good documentation is a skill that is almost as necessary as good patient care.

- Your medical report may be subpoenaed for a criminal or civil action, and an attorney may subpoena you as well to testify as to the events in question.
- Civil actions often take up to 7 years to reach a jury trial, which would mean you would have to recount facts 7 years after they occurred.
- You may remember inserting an oropharyngeal airway, but if the written report of the event consists solely of "no breathing, started CPR," then the attorney will present to the jury that the OPA was perhaps never inserted.

Good Documentation Is Good Patient Care

As an EMT, you are often the first medical provider to interact with a patient, thus your observations may be critical in the patient's course of treatment. The physician who ultimately becomes responsible for a patient's care will have been far removed from the initial point of care. The PCR may be the only way the physician can picture the situation that brought the patient to her care.

Let's say you arrive on the scene of a "man down" call. The patient is a 40-year-old male who is actively seizing with his hands clenched and rotated inward. As you reach the patient's side, the seizure subsides, his hands relax to a normal position, and he is now unconscious. There is no indication of trauma, so you perform an initial assessment that is unremarkable. The bystanders are not aware of any medical history. You transport to the nearest emergency department, and en route the patient begins to regain consciousness but is confused and disoriented. His vitals remain stable, and as you discharge him to the emergency department he is becoming more lucid. By the time the physician sees him, he may have completely returned to normal, with no memory of the events that brought him to the hospital.

The EMT's PCR in this case is crucial to the patient's treatment, especially if decorticate posturing (hands clenched and rotated inward) was noted, a possible indication of brain injury.

Run Report or "Charting"

The run report will contain the following information:

- Current date
- Patient's name, address, phone number
- Gender
- Date of birth and possibly a Social Security/insurance number (not required by all services)
- Medical history
- Current medications and known allergies
- Narrative of events and treatment
  - Gives the story of the encounter and paints a picture that will allow the reader to visualize what you saw and experienced
  - Provides the context for why you took the actions you did in treating and transporting the patient
  - Includes any findings made during the patient assessments, including baseline vital signs
  - States clearly and definitively the chief complaint
  - Includes specific patient comments on scene in quotation marks, such as "I had too much to drink," which should be put in quotation marks
  - May include some abbreviations as governed by local medical usage
- Patient's and provider's signatures

The run report is a confidential medical document. Completed run reports must be secured and not left out where they can be read by anyone nearby. If a run report is used for training or educational purposes, you must remove any information that could identify the patient.

Since the PCR is a legal document, it should state only the actual facts of a call as the EMT records them. False statements on the run report—including omissions of protocol steps—should never be made and could have several serious consequences:

- Could place you in danger of losing your license or certification to practice
- Could open the service (and potentially you) to increased legal liability, including possible criminal charges
- Could cause the patient to be given inappropriate follow-up care at the receiving facility, with possible adverse effects

If any error is made on the paper PCR, any corrections must be noted and signed. This is usually accomplished by placing a horizontal line through the incorrect information and then noting the date and time of the correction with the initials of the report writer.

If utilizing an ePCR format, information may be deleted and rewritten just as you would on a computer, as long as the run report has not been submitted as final yet. If the run report has been submitted as final yet the EMT needs to correct a mistake or omission, either an addendum can be attached to the chart or the chart can be "reopened" by a supervisor.

Patient refusal issues are increasingly problematic to EMS, so the documentation of refusals must be especially thorough. Proceed as follows:

- An adult patient of sound mind can refuse medical treatment or transport. If you believe that a specific treatment or hospital transport is appropriate, you must explain the rationale to the patient; if the patient continues to refuse, you must document both your explanation and the patient's refusal.

- Your documentation should include a note that the patient was informed of the potential consequence of not following the EMT's recommendations.

- Once the documentation is complete, have the patient sign the refusal, witnessed by an impartial third party (ideally a police officer if one is on scene).

- If the patient refuses to sign the release, then ask an impartial third party to witness that you explained the procedures and consequences.

In addition to the PCR, you must also be familiar with the written documents in use by your service. These reports will include injury reports for EMS personnel in the line of duty, auto accident reports following incidents involving the EMS vehicle, infectious disease-exposure reports, and police witness statements if you have witnessed a criminal act or are the victim of a crime. Any of these reports should be attached to the PCR for the incident during which they occurred, as well as placed in the appropriate personnel and service files.

Many states and services require that a run report, whether on paper or electronic, be completed and submitted within 24 hours of the completed call. (In fact, some services require submission of a run report before you are allowed to take a new 911 call.) Get in the habit of doing your reporting quickly and neatly.

TEST YOURSELF 4.3

Can this patient refuse care?

You are dispatched to an unknown medical call but are told that the bystander caller states the patient is "confused." Upon arrival, you find a 32-year-old male who is stumbling around the living room and slurring his words; however, he is cooperative when asked to take a seat. BP is 128/72 mm Hg, respiratory rate is 14/min, and pulse rate is 92. Blood sugar level is 68 mg/dL. He states that he does not want to go to the hospital. He is able to answer your questions, but at a slower rate than normal. His friend states he is a known diabetic.

After oral glucose administration, his blood sugar rises to 76. He still slurs his words, but he is becoming more clear. He still does not want to go to the hospital. Does he have the right to refuse care at this point?

Practice Set

1. You respond with lights and sirens to assist the police at a domestic violence incident. You arrive on scene and observe two police cars with their lights flashing in the driveway and a female lying prone on the lawn in front of the residence. You hear gunfire coming from the residence. Your correct course of action is which of the following?

    A. Request additional rescues immediately

    B. Rush to the female, stabilize her cervical spine, and check her airway

    C. Withdraw your unit from the residence

    D. Enter the dwelling to check for additional victims while your partner assists the female in the yard

2. You respond to a fight in progress. The police advise the scene is secure, and you are wearing suitable protective equipment. Your patient is a male, thirty-ish, seated on the steps of a residence, bent over and clutching his chest. He is making noisy respiratory sounds and is groaning in pain. You can smell the odor of alcohol. You check his carotid pulse, and he has a good pulse with a rate of 80. There are no signs of gross hemorrhage. Your next step is to perform which of the following assessments?

    A. Focused medical assessment

    B. Focused trauma assessment

    C. Initial assessment

    D. Medical insurance assessment

3. You are dispatched to a motorcycle accident on the freeway. You respond emergently and arrive on scene. You observe three police cars on scene, a destroyed motorcycle lying on its side, and a man lying supine next to the motorcycle with a large piece of the front fork of the motorcycle sticking out of his abdomen. The scene is safe and you are wearing suitable protection. You approach the patient, and the next thing you do is which of the following?

    A. Check his airway

    B. Stabilize the large piece of metal with cravats and bandages

    C. Request a physician to the scene to perform a surgical removal

    D. Transfer the patient to a backboard and transport immediately

4. You arrive on scene to find a patient lying supine on the ground. As you approach the patient, you can hear him breathing and observe his chest rising and falling. The scene is secure, and you are wearing appropriate protective equipment. His eyes are closed, and you shake his shoulder and ask his name. He has no response. You shout at him asking if he's all right, and his eyes open and he groans. You ask him what happened, and he does not appear to understand at all. You rub his sternum, and he yells, "Ow!" Which of the following best describes his level of consciousness?

    A. Conscious and alert

    B. Responsive to pain

    C. Responsive to verbal

    D. Unresponsive

5. You are called to a residence for a man down, possibly intoxicated. The police have secured the scene by the time you arrive. There are no bystanders. You are wearing proper protective clothing. You observe a large male lying on the floor next to the couch. He is breathing and has a carotid pulse. There is no gross hemorrhage, and his capillary refill is approximately 5 seconds. What condition should you suspect?

   A. Intoxication

   B. Circulatory compromise

   C. Respiratory distress

   D. Heroin overdose

6. Which of the following patients would be given a priority transport?

   A. Female in second-stage labor

   B. 18-year-old male with a suspected radius fracture from falling during a soccer game

   C. 12-year-old female with difficulty breathing and a history of asthma

   D. 2-year-old male who fell out of his crib and is crying loudly

7. Which of the following patients would be given a priority transport?

   A. Male patient conscious and alert with a blood pressure of 210/110 mm Hg

   B. Female patient in labor with respiratory rate of 20/minute

   C. Male patient with a pulse rate of 110/minute

   D. Female patient with a pulse rate of 20/minute

8. Who can answer the SAMPLE questions for a conscious, alert adult patient assessment?

   A. Police

   B. Bystanders

   C. Your partner

   D. The patient

9. Which of the following conditions noted during the focused trauma assessment would indicate immediate transport?

   A. Unconscious

   B. Low blood sugar

   C. Tracheal shift to right

   D. Pedestrian struck by car on city street

10. You are dispatched for a bicyclist struck by a car. On your arrival, your patient is lying supine on the ground, not moving. You approach your patient from the feet, take manual stabilization of his head, and check his airway. He is breathing and you can palpate a carotid pulse, which appears rapid. You ask in a loud voice if he is okay and get no response. Your partner rubs the patient's sternum with his thumb and your patient opens his eyes, groans, and moves his hand to his chest to push your partner's hand away. There is a large bruise with swelling on the right side of his head and no other apparent injuries. His vital signs are BP 160/100 mm Hg, pulse 60/min, and respirations 15/min. What would be his revised trauma score?

    A. 8

    B. 9

    C. 10

    D. 11

11. You arrive on the scene of an MVA, car vs. pole. Your patient is a 25-year-old female who was ejected from her vehicle when it struck a telephone pole. The car is totally demolished. Your initial assessment is that your patient is unconscious and unresponsive. Due to the MOI and patient ejection, you determine that this is a "load and go," immobilize your patient, and begin transport. As you do your focused trauma assessment, you notice that the patient's left upper quadrant is now rigid, whereas in the initial assessment it appeared normal. What should be your next action?

    A. Nothing, continue with the assessment and see what else comes up injury wise

    B. Place a non-rebreather mask at 6 liter per minute on the patient's face

    C. Request your driver to expedite as you suspect your patient has an intra-abdominal bleed

    D. Perform a modified jaw thrust

12. You are dispatched to a report of a female intoxicated. The scene is secure and you are wearing suitable precautions. You arrive on scene and find a female in her forties lying supine, unconscious, and responsive (groans) to painful stimuli. You detect an odor of alcohol, and her friend confirms heavy drinking all evening. There is no indication of trauma, and your initial assessment is unremarkable. You place the patient in the truck, administer 10 liters oxygen via non-rebreather mask, and begin priority transport to the nearest emergency department 15 minutes away. You notify the hospital of the patient's condition and vital signs. After disconnecting from the hospital, you begin to reassess your patient and now notice that she is not breathing. Your next step is which of the following?

    A. Advise the driver to expedite

    B. Insert an oropharyngeal airway and ventilate at 10–12 times per minute

    C. Continue the assessment to try and discover any other conditions

    D. Retake pulse, respiratory rate, and blood pressure

13. If the patient tells you that his symptoms started 20 minutes ago, what letter is this represented by in the mnemonic OPQRST?

    A. Time

    B. Events leading up to situation

    C. Onset

    D. Estimated time of arrival

14. What do the letters B and P stand for in the mnemonic DCAP-BTLS?

    A. Burn, puncture

    B. Bruise, pain

    C. Bruise, penetration

    D. Burn, pain

15. You are dispatched to a call for a 34-year-old fall victim. Upon arrival at the scene, you note that the patient has a strong odor of alcohol on his breath and there are multiple beer bottles on the table near where he is sitting. His girlfriend is the person who called 911 and states that he was drinking and tripped on the rug and fell onto the table, striking his head. She states that he did not have any loss of consciousness, and you do not see any major bleeding from the patient's head. The patient does not wish to transport to the hospital, saying, "I'm fine. She shouldn't have called," and is slurring his words. What is your next step?

    A. Get your partner to take a baseline set of vitals and as long as they are in the normal range, have him sign a refusal and leave the scene

    B. Call for police backup as you may have to take the patient to your ambulance forcefully

    C. Explain that due to his level of inebriation and the fact that he struck his head, he is unfortunately not able to refuse at this time, and it would be in his best interest to come to the hospital for evaluation

    D. Say okay, have the girlfriend sign the refusal form, and leave the patient in her care

16. When completing a refusal form on a conscious, alert, and oriented × 4 competent adult patient, who should sign the refusal form?

    A. Only the patient

    B. The patient and their spouse

    C. The patient and an impartial third party such as a police officer on scene

    D. The patient and their 17-year-old son or daughter

17. Falsification of a run report can result in the following?

    A. Nothing, as long as it was never submitted in the first place

    B. Arrest of the EMT and jail time up to 7 years

    C. Incorrect care of the patient at the hospital

    D. Possible legal action, loss of right to practice as an EMT, and possible damage to the patient with follow-up care

18. You arrive on the scene of a one-car motor vehicle accident. The car left the lane of travel and struck the soft shoulder, where it appears to have rolled over at least once. The driver is a female, approximate age 40, who is conscious, alert, and oriented × 4. Your partner applies head stabilization from the backseat while you conduct the assessment. The patient states that she's fine and just wants a ride to the hospital. The windshield is cracked, and the patient is not wearing a seat belt. She has a bruise on the front of her forehead. You explain that you want to apply a cervical collar and then a Kendrick™ Extrication Device (KED) to remove her from the vehicle to protect her spine. She becomes agitated and announces that all she wants is a ride to the hospital, nothing more. She begins to get out of the car. Which of the following options is most appropriate?

    A. Let her walk herself to the truck and transport her to the hospital

    B. Notify her that the police will place her in protective custody and then you will be able to do whatever you want

    C. Explain to her the risks of spinal injury unless you take the proper precautions and, if she continues to refuse, fill out a narrative documenting your explanation and her refusal and have her sign it in the presence of the police

    D. Disregard her protests and apply the cervical collar and KED

19. You respond to a call from the police station for a male with chest pains. You respond emergently with appropriate BSI precautions. You arrive on scene and find a male in his forties seated in a chair clutching his chest, in obvious distress. He is pale, diaphoretic, and having difficulty breathing. There is no indication of trauma. He states that he's fine and refuses all treatment and transport options. He is not in police custody, but is the victim of a crime. Which of the following options is most appropriate?

    A. Explain the consequences of his refusal and have him sign the refusal form, witnessed by a police officer

    B. Disregard his objections, administer oxygen via non-rebreather, and transport priority to the nearest hospital emergency department

    C. Patiently explain the seriousness of his condition and continue to encourage him to allow you to treat him and transport him to the hospital

    D. When his eyes are closed, administer nitroglycerin sublingual

20. A patient becomes unconscious as you are trying to get him to agree to go to the hospital. He has never given you permission for treatment or transport, so your next move would be which of the following?

    A. Initiate appropriate treatment under the doctrine of implied consent

    B. Document that the patient never gave permission to treat, note that the patient is now unconscious and cannot sign the refusal, and have a police officer sign verifying your explanation

    C. Transport the patient priority, but do not perform any treatments since you do not have the patient's permission

    D. Initiate appropriate treatment in accordance with local protocols under the doctrine of expressed consent

Answers and Explanations

1.   C

The scene is not safe, and you should not be there. You can request additional rescues (A) at any time. Your primary inclination may be to run to the female (B), but you run the risk of becoming a victim yourself. Entering a dwelling from which you hear gunfire (D) is incredibly dangerous and may result in you or your partner being shot.

2.   C

The temptation is to answer (B), as this is most probably a trauma, but taking shortcuts compromises the EMT's ability to make the correct determinations. An initial assessment covers the ABCs first, regardless of how the potential injury or illness happened. The noisy respirations are a cause for concern and need to be addressed before a more focused assessment and head-to-toe exam should be done.

3.   A

Even though this is a "load and go" situation due to the magnitude of the patient's injuries, a patient without an airway will arrive at the ER dead. If the patient has a patent airway, is breathing, and has a pulse, then stabilize the metal (B) and prepare for immediate transport. Requesting a physician to the scene (C) would take too much time and would endanger the patient more. The metal can be removed best in an operating room.

4.   C

When assessing for level of responsiveness, take the BEST and highest level of response the patient has. Here, the patient did not respond to normal stimuli, so he is not conscious and alert (A). The next level is verbal (C), and this is where he responded by opening his eyes and groaning when you shouted his name. While he also responded to pain toward the end, the higher level (verbal) would apply, as he did initially respond to your shouting. Finally, as he responded to both verbal and pain, he would not be considered unresponsive (D).

5.   B

This is a challenging question and the quick answer without performing a complete assessment is (A). However, other than the dispatch there are no indicators in your primary physical or scene assessment that indicate alcohol intoxication. The fact that the patient's nail beds take so long to return to pink would indicate that his circulation is impaired. While respiratory compromise and heroin overdose are possibilities, circulatory compromise is the better answer.

6.   C

While all the choices are possibilities if secondary assessment finds something significant or conditions change, the patient with difficulty breathing needs to be expedited. The ABCs must always be addressed first.

7.   D

A patient with a pulse of 20/min will present with symptoms of low perfusion, including pale skin and diminished level of consciousness. The other vital signs may be out of normal range, but in the absence of a life-threatening condition would be considered a non-priority transport.

8.   D

The clue here is that the patient is conscious, alert, and an adult. Unless you suspect that the patient's mental status is compromised, the patient should always be the first source of information for your SAMPLE questions. In the absence of a compromised mental status (or suspicion of one), bystanders or family members may be able to provide some information. Obtaining answers becomes even more problematic when the patient is unconscious or incoherent.

9. C

Tracheal shift to either side is indicative of a tension pneumothorax, a collapsed lung that is pushing against other organs and may lead to other organ failure or damage. It can be relieved only by a chest tube, which is beyond the scope of the EMT. (A) is a condition that should have been found in the initial assessment and by itself does not indicate immediate transport. Neither does (B), which can be treated by the EMT in the field in some services or by calling for an ALS assist. A pedestrian struck (D) has a high incidence of suspicion due to the nature of the injury, but, again, by itself is not indicative of an immediate transport.

10. D

The first thing you must calculate is the Glasgow Coma Scale. His eyes open to pain, giving him a 2; his words are incomprehensible, giving him a 2; and he localizes pain, which gives him a 5. So total GCS is 9, making the trauma score index a 3. In calculating the trauma score, he gets 4 for respiratory rate between 10 and 29, 4 for having a systolic blood pressure greater than 89, and 3 for the GCS, which gives him a trauma score of 11. Use care in calculating mathematical questions like this, since one of your choices is 9, which is the GCS. It's always a good idea to run calculations twice to be sure.

11. C

While you suspected a serious injury before, the development of a rigid left upper quadrant is fairly indicative of a ruptured spleen, which will result in the patient's bleeding intra-abdominally. The only treatment for this condition is removal of the spleen in an operating room. Doing nothing (A) is inappropriate because you must realize this is an injury that will benefit the most by getting the patient to a hospital sooner rather than later. Your goal is getting this patient to an operating room as soon as possible. (B) is not the appropriate liters per minute to be used with a non-rebreather mask. (D) should have already been done on the scene, not at this time.

12. B

A patient needs oxygen to live, and if she is not breathing then she will die. The airway must first be secured and then the patient ventilated. You can advise the driver to expedite once this is taken care of. (C) and (D) can be undertaken if you have another EMT in the back of the truck, but if you are alone your concern must be for the patient's airway and respirations.

13. C

Onset is when the symptoms started, while time (A) is how long the symptoms have been occurring or whether the patient has experienced this type of symptom before. (B) is part of the SAMPLE questions, and (D) is used when giving a prehospital radio report.

14. A

While P stands for either puncture or penetration, none of the other answers give the correct answer in its entirety.

15. C

Unfortunately, due to the patient's level of intoxication, strong odor of alcohol on his breath, slurred words, the scene survey of multiple bottles of beer next to him, as well as the head strike, this patient is considered not competent to make an educated decision about his transport. Leaving this patient in his home could lead to further complications such as a head bleed or worse, death. Having him sign a refusal at this point would also put the EMT in a precarious position if this chart would ever go to court. The EMT may need to call for police backup (B), but that would be only after trying to convince the patient to go himself (unless there were some type of danger involved).

16. C

The correct answer is (C) because it is the most legally protective. The third party is impartial. A family member may not be impartial, but note that some systems may allow (B) to happen if there is no other suitable option; this should be used as a last resort. (D) is incorrect due to the fact that the witness is underage.

17. D

The EMT should never falsify the run report for any reason at any time. If an honest mistake is made in charting, whether it is electronic or written, the proper correction method must be used. Doing nothing (A) is a bad mindset. Arrest and jail time (B) is not always true. Incorrect patient care (C) may happen but not always. Choice (D) is the broadest answer of what could happen.

18. C

(C) describes the appropriate course of action in this matter. (A) is wrong because you have not yet documented your explanation and treatment options, and if she persists, you may become liable for injuries. (B) is wrong because unless the police have probable cause for placing the person in protective custody, they will not do it. (D) may be considered assault and battery.

19. C

The potential seriousness of the situation really requires you to stand by as long as possible. (A) is legally correct, but if the patient's condition changes as soon as you drive out of the parking lot, a jury might consider it abandonment. (B) is assault and battery, and possibly kidnapping. (D) is also assault, since you do not have the patient's permission to give treatment, even if it is allowed by your protocols.

20. A

Implied consent means that an unconscious patient would want you to treat him if he were conscious, even if he initially declined. This doctrine is well established in case law. (B) is abandonment, (C) is as well, and (D) is incorrect because expressed consent would be the patient agreeing to your treatment and transport recommendations, which this patient never did.

CHAPTER 5

Respiratory Emergencies and Airway Management

Topics Discussed

- **Respiratory Emergencies and How They Happen**
- **Conducting a Proper Respiratory Assessment**
- **Opening the Airway**
- **Airway Adjuncts**
- **Artificial Centilation Techniques and Oxygen Delivery Systems**

In order to live and breathe, every patient needs an airway, a pathway for oxygen to travel from the outside environment to the alveoli, where it can enter the bloodstream to be used in the metabolic process. If any part of this pathway is interrupted somehow, via a disease process or trauma to its structures, it becomes incredibly difficult for the person to breathe, if at all. The EMT must be able to recognize when a respiratory emergency is happening and take decisive, quick steps to remedy the situation or else they will soon have a deceased patient on their hands.

How Respiratory Emergencies Happen

In a normal, healthy person, air flow is a continuous cycle of oxygenated air that is brought in through the oropharynx and nasopharynx and introduced into the lungs by the act of respiration and ventilation.

Remember that **respiration** is the act of gas exchange of oxygen and carbon dioxide that happens at the capillary level. This is different from the act of **ventilation**, which is the movement of air in and out of something—either the body or through artificial means such as a bag-valve-mask device.

When there is an interruption of the air flow or gas exchange at any level or structure in the respiratory system, the body will become distressed. The brain's respiratory centers located in the brainstem will recognize that there is an issue and trigger the body to either speed up or slow down the person's breathing pattern depending on the situation at hand. When the burden becomes too great for the person to handle on their own, this is when emergency services are called. In fact, respiratory distress is one of the most common EMS calls you will receive.

The EMT must be able to recognize not only the different levels of distress a person can experience, but also the possibilities of WHY the emergency is happening so that swift action can be taken.

The different levels of respiratory emergencies are distress, failure, and arrest.

Distress is when the person is experiencing **tachypnea** (fast breathing), **bradypnea** (slow breathing), or an obstruction of some sort. This is the level where your quick actions can prevent a further downfall for the patient.

- They may be in a tripod position or have pillows propping them up, as it is more difficult to breath while laying supine.
- They may have difficulty speaking in full sentences.
- They may have a lowered pulse oximeter (SpO2) reading.
- They may start to have some color changes in their skin.
- Their capillary refill time may be delayed and take more than 2 seconds to return to normal.
- They may already be or start to get very anxious—this could be a result of **hypoxia,** or low levels of oxygen in their blood.

Failure can be either an acute or chronic condition in which not enough oxygen passes from the lungs into the bloodstream or when the lungs can't properly remove carbon dioxide from the blood. Too much carbon dioxide in the blood can harm the body's organs.

- In acute cases, these people will need ventilatory support or they will quickly progress into the final stage of arrest.
- In chronic cases, they will oftentimes be on home oxygen or use various medications to manage their condition and have a baseline lower level of oxygen saturation rates.
- They may display "pursed lips breathing," in which they breathe in through their nose, then exhale through puckered lips. The lips look as if they are trying to kiss something or someone. This helps to create pressure to keep the airways open and may be done consciously or subconsciously.

Arrest is when the body ceases to breathe properly on its own. These people absolutely need artificial ventilatory support done by the EMT. Oftentimes the heart will soon cease to beat as well shortly after if respiratory function is not restored.

- Color changes in the skin will range from gray to blue to white.
- Be prepared to perform CPR if necessary.

So now that you can recognize some warning signs of the various levels of respiratory emergencies, let's review how to do a proper assessment.

Respiratory Assessment

To properly assess respiratory function, the EMT must note the following signs or symptoms:

- Observe the rise and fall of the chest as the patient breathes
- Look for accessory muscle usage, particularly in the neck and intercostal spaces

- Check body positioning, i.e., is the patient tripoding or propped up?
- Check for adequate volume, i.e., is the patient breathing deeply or taking shallow breaths?
- Listen for speech, i.e., is the patient speaking in full sentences without difficulty or are breaths required in between words?
- Measure oxygen saturation (SpO2) level using a pulse oximeter
- Auscultate (listen by stethoscope) the lungs

From this list, there are three items that require further clarification: checking for breath sounds, measuring oxygen saturation, and checking for an open airway.

Checking the airway should always be done first to see if any obstruction is occurring that would need to be relieved. Remember that if a patient is able to speak to you in full sentences without distress, they most likely have an open airway. To efficiently use time wisely, you may place the pulse oximeter onto the patient's finger and wait for it to calculate while you attempt to listen to lung sounds.

Checking for Breath Sounds

Textbooks differ on the best locations to listen for breath sounds. Since there are five lung lobes or sections—three on the right and two on the left—a comprehensive assessment should include them all. The best way to do so is to locate the following six anatomical landmarks and place a stethoscope on them.

- Left chest, proximal to the clavicle at the midclavicular line: listen for the breath sound, which should be the sound of air flowing in and out without obstruction
- Right chest, proximal to the clavicle at the midclavicular line: always listen to one side and then the other (bilateral auscultation) to compare the sounds in opposite fields
- Left lateral chest on the midaxillary line
- Right lateral chest on the midaxillary line
- Left back below the scapula, opposite the midclavicular line
- Right back below the scapula, opposite the midclavicular line

Abnormal (or *adventitious*) breath sounds can be a major clue for the EMT to understand not only why the patient is breathing a certain way but also how to proceed with the treatment.

The EMT must be able to identify the following sounds. If you are struggling with telling the difference, review the sounds in a multimedia library online.

- **Crackles/rales**: rattling, crackling, clinking, or popping noises; label "fine" or "coarse" to indicate the loudness with which they can be heard
  - Caused by fluid in the small airway passages or collapsed alveoli
  - Can be heard on both inspiration and expiration
  - Occur when the smaller airways open suddenly during inspiration

- **Wheezes**: squeaky, musical, or moan-like noises
  - Caused by air moving through airways narrowed by constriction, swelling of the airway, partial airway obstruction, or excess secretions
  - Can be heard on expiration in early stages, but on inspiration and expiration as the airways become more compromised
- **Pleural friction rubs**: low-pitched, grating, or creaking sounds (as when sitting down on a leather couch)
  - Caused by inflamed pleural lung surfaces rubbing together during respiration
  - Can be heard on both inspiration and expiration
- **Stridor**: high-pitched, almost whistle-like sound
  - Caused by obstruction or blockage of the upper airway, e.g., object or inflammation of upper airway anatomical structures such as epiglottis
  - Can be heard on inspiration
- **Rhonchi**: low-pitched clunky or rattling sounds, even snore-like in quality
  - Caused by obstruction or buildup of mucus in large airways
  - Often cleared with coughing

Once you understand how to conduct a respiratory assessment, you need to know the signs and symptoms of adequate (and inadequate) breathing. The four criteria for this are *rate, rhythm, quality*, and *tidal volume*.

- **Rate**: the term "normal" is always subject to debate and textbooks differ on what is a normal adult respiratory rate, some stating 8–24 respirations per minute and others 12–20. If we average out the two, a rate higher than 22 would be considered tachypnea, and a rate lower than 9 would be considered bradypnea.
- **Rhythm** is determined by noting the times of inspiration, exhalation, and pause between. They should be equal between each cycle.
- **Quality** is determined by use of the accessory muscles. If the patient is utilizing the accessory muscles of the intercostal spaces and neck in order to breathe, or is having some type of difficulty, then it must be noted.
- **Tidal volume** (or depth of ventilation) must be sufficient for the person to speak normally, and the chest should rise and fall with each breath cycle.

If everything appears to be within a normal range and does not raise any red flags, the EMT can then move on to assessing the next part of the body. However, if the airway is not **patent** (open), the patient is in distress, or ventilatory assistance is required, the EMT must continuing exploring WHY and fix problems here before moving on with the assessment.

Measuring Oxygen Saturation

To measure oxygen saturation, the EMT uses a pulse oximeter, a noninvasive tool that measures the amount of oxygen being carried in the body.

It is helpful in determining the patient's need for oxygen, and how best to deliver it.

- Types include handheld monitor, separate corded unit on a cardiac monitor, or fingertip-only unit with a built-in screen.
- Sends 2 wavelengths of light through the finger to measure both the pulse rate and amount of oxygen in the body system.
- Once the oximeter finishes its assessment, the screen will display the percentage of oxygen.

Generally, oxygen saturation for a normal, healthy patient should be 94–100%. Anything <94% oxygen saturation should be explored and potentially corrected, but keep in mind that certain patients live with a baseline of lowered saturation rates, so be sure to do a whole assessment and ask good questions.

Be careful to monitor the patient and not just the pulse oximeter. If the patient is not presenting in any respiratory distress, take the whole picture into account. Treat the patient, not the equipment.

Check for things such as nail polish on the hands/feet, cold hands, incorrect placement of the oximeter on the finger, and even low batteries on the machine. Any of these situations can skew a true oximeter reading.

Checking for an Open Airway

The EMT's first concern with an occluded or blocked airway is to open it to enable the patient to breathe. Assuming you have deemed a scenario safe and are wearing the proper protective equipment, do the following:

1. Approach the patient (usually from the feet if patient is lying down) and scan the area for anything that may indicate a change in the scene status or that may have caused the emergency to which you are responding.
2. If there is no response, kneel at the patient's head and hold the cervical spine in place. Bend down over the patient's nose and mouth to see if you can hear breathing sounds or feel exhalations on your cheek. Watch the patient's chest to see if there is any breathing motion.
3. If these signs are negative, your next move must be to open the patient's airway.

Opening the patient's airway is a lifesaving maneuver. It involves your being able to diagnose an occluded airway and then use both gloved hands to open and clear the oropharynx to let air into the trachea.

Trauma Considerations

If you suspect a traumatic event, the most important concerns are to stabilize the neck and provide an open airway and breathing. Using the jaw-thrust maneuver is the most appropriate way to minimize cervical movement while still achieving an open airway.

Be aware that you may need another EMT to complete the rest of the body assessment while you continue to secure the airway. Be sure spinal precautions have been properly taken and a properly sized cervical collar (c-collar) has been secured to the patient.

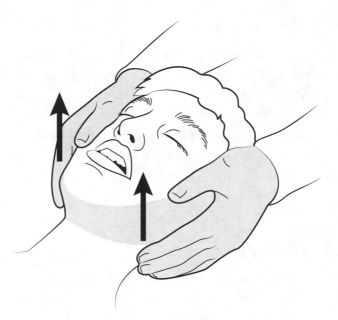

Figure 5.1 *Jaw-Thrust Maneuver*

The purpose of the jaw-thrust maneuver is to minimize cervical spine movement, including stabilization of the neck and providing an open airway for breathing. Any other problems that may be noted should be addressed later.

- Hold the patient's head and place your ring and little fingers underneath the head, with your thumbs alongside the head.
- Place your first and middle fingers of both hands beneath the jawbone (mandible) and push upward. This action will lift not only the mandible, but also the tongue—which is attached to the structures of the mouth—by pulling the tongue away from the posterior larynx.
- Look into the mouth to see if there is anything physically blocking it (if there is, have your partner remove it) and begin artificial respirations if they do not begin spontaneously.

Non-Trauma Considerations

If you have ruled out or do not suspect a trauma scenario, the actions are essentially the same, except that the airway can be opened by using the head-tilt, chin-lift method.

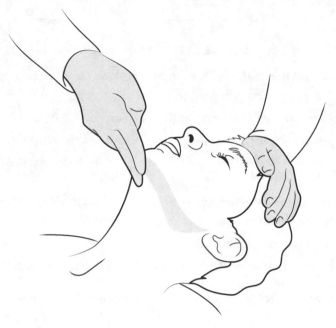

Figure 5.2 *Head-Tilt, Chin-Lift Maneuver*

To do this maneuver, do the following:

- Lift the chin using the first and middle fingers and push the forehead back. This will move the tongue away from the posterior larynx.

- Maintain this position by placing a rolled towel/blanket underneath the patient's shoulders, which will allow you to have your hands free.

- If the airway is blocked by solids, clear it by removing the object (assuming it can be seen) by using forceps. The EMT may also elect to do chest compressions to try and relieve the unseen object as per the most recent AHA guidelines if the person is unresponsive or was known to be choking prior to becoming unresponsive. If the airway is blocked by fluids such as vomit, then suctioning may be indicated.

Suctioning the Airway

If the EMT determines that there is a solid or fluid obstruction to the airway, suction may be indicated and should be used early on. Be aware that **aspiration**, or the movement of fluids or solids, can occur where they move farther down into the trachea or to the lungs.

Suction units come in both handheld non-electric and electric/battery-powered models. Most EMS units carry both, so it is up to you to make sure you know where and how your equipment works prior to going on your first call of the shift.

If an EMT does not have a working suction unit available in the field, it could have devastating consequences for a patient. Check your equipment at the beginning of every shift.

There are two types of suction catheter: hard tip (or Yankauer) and soft, flexible tip.

- **Hard-tipped suction catheter** (Yankauer) is designed to allow effective suction without damaging surrounding tissue.
  - Firm plastic with large opening at the end, surrounded by bulbous head
  - Appropriate for most scenarios, except for cases of clenched teeth or where the EMT cannot fit the suction tip in the orifice to be suctioned (e.g., tracheostomy or nostrils)
- **Soft-tipped suction catheter** is more flexible; it comes in various sizes that can be inserted via the mouth or nose, or through a tracheostomy port.
  - Latex-free material, flexible, with a small diameter
  - Appropriate for more challenging scenarios, e.g., clenched teeth

No matter the type of catheter you use, the steps for **suctioning the mouth** remain the same.

1. Make sure proper PPE is on (this includes gloves and protective glasses in case of splatter of bodily fluids). Aprons should also be made available.
2. Open the airway using the proper technique (trauma vs. non) and visualize the airway to see if suctioning is needed.
3. Select the proper suction catheter and attach it to the suction tubing that is on a working suction unit.
4. Turn on the unit if indicated (hand-powered models do not have a power button and rely on a squeezing motion to work).
5. Place the suction catheter tip into the patient's mouth no farther than the base of the tongue.
6. Place your finger over the designated vent hole on the suction catheter in order to create the vacuum seal.
7. Suction for no more than 10–15 seconds on the way OUT of the mouth using a back and forth motion to get to all corners of the mouth.
8. Remove the catheter from the mouth and clear the tip by suctioning up a small amount of water to "flush" the catheter out.
9. Repeat the steps above as necessary to clear the oropharynx.

Never suction for more than 10–15 seconds at a time, since the suctioning also removes oxygen from the oropharynx.

Suctioning a tracheostomy tube is similar to the steps listed above, however a soft-tipped catheter tip is more appropriately sized for the opening of the tube. Insert the suction catheter into the tracheostomy until resistance is felt, then pull back about 1/2 inch. Use the same concept of no more than 10–15 seconds at a time of suction, as you will also be removing oxygen from the patient's system.

Suctioning the nasopharynx calls for use of a soft-tipped suction tip and requires you to lubricate the tip prior to insertion. The steps above are similar to the process here with the exception that if the patient is conscious, it is suggested to keep the patient at a 45-degree angle to help facilitate the process. Once the tip is lubricated, advance the catheter tip until a gag reflex is induced or resistance is met and use the same principles as listed above to suction the airway.

Airway Adjuncts

There will be cases when you will need to insert an airway adjunct in order to maintain a patent airway and ensure proper oxygenation. Airway adjuncts come in both adult and pediatric sizes.

Oropharyngeal Airway

An oropharyngeal airway (OPA) is a device hooked underneath the tongue, which holds it away from the posterior larynx. Various shapes and sizes are available.

- Measured for length by measuring from the tip of the ear to the corner of the mouth
- Inserted backward (rotated 180 degrees) to the normal anatomical position and twisted into position
- Alternatively, inserted in anatomical position as a tongue depressor holds down the tongue while OPA is moved into position behind the tongue; if patient gags during insertion, withdraw immediately and use another method

Nasopharyngeal Airway

A nasopharyngeal airway (NPA) holds the nasopharynx open and lifts the tongue, with the use of a soft tube inserted into the nasopharynx through the nose.

- Can be used on patients with a gag reflex or whose teeth are clenched because of seizure or some other medical condition
- Measured for length by measuring from the tip of the patient's nose to the tip of the ear
- Lubricated with sterile water-soluble lubricant and inserted into the larger nostril with the bevel toward the septum with a back-and-forth twisting motion; once the flange of the NPA reaches the nostril, stop inserting and evaluate your patient
- Contraindicated in patients with facial trauma or possible skull fracture, as there may be an opening that would allow the NPA to enter the cranial compartment

What airway tools would you use with this patient?

Your patient is a 19-year-old female who was driving home after a party and smashed her car into a tree. She had been drinking heavily. Her friend, who was a passenger in the car, self-extricated and is now being assessed by your partner. Your patient says, "I think my nose is broken" and then coughs up some blood, which is bright red. She faints at the sight of this and collapses to the ground, hitting legs first. You immediately check a pulse, which is found to be present. You notice a large amount of blood leaking from the mouth and note her breathing rate to be at 10.

Which airway opening maneuver should you use and why? What type of suction tip would you use? What airway adjunct would you use?

Respiratory Emergencies

The severity of respiratory emergencies can range from simple dyspnea to apnea (cessation of respiratory function). This section will discuss the more common respiratory diseases.

This is a good time to review the anatomy and physiology of the respiratory system, which is necessary to recognize and treat the various conditions that come under this heading.

Dyspnea

One of the most common EMS dispatches is for difficulty breathing (dyspnea). The causes and manifestations of this broad-based condition include conditions such as asthma, bronchitis, and emphysema.

The signs and symptoms of dyspnea may include any of the following:

- Shortness of breath (SOB), restlessness, increased pulse rate, changes in respiratory rate (>20 or <12 breaths/min in adults)
- Changes in skin color (bluish gray, pale, or flushed)
- Noisy respirations (wheezing, gurgling, snoring, or stridor)
- Inability to speak

- Breathing that uses accessory muscles or the abdomen or breathing that has an irregular rhythm
- Altered mental status
- Patient in tripod position (hunched forward with arms rotated outward) and barrel chest

Emergency Care of Dyspnea

If the patient is conscious and able to answer questions, the OPQRST (Onset, Provocation, Quality, Radiation, Severity, Time of onset) questions are appropriate at this time. These are then followed by the SAMPLE (Signs and symptoms, Allergies, Medications, Past history, Last oral intake, and Events leading to this condition) questions.

In addition to these questions, if the patient indicates that she has an inhaler or uses some other intervention, then you want to ask if she has used one of these interventions since the onset of this set of symptoms and whether or not there was any change in her condition as a result. If the patient is unconscious or unable to speak, then a family member or other bystander may have to be the source for this information.

If the patient is unconscious, the EMT must take swift steps to secure the airway and be ready to deliver artificial ventilations if necessary.

If the patient is conscious, follow the steps below to both assess and treat a patient experiencing dyspnea:

1. Take a set of baseline vitals, including pulse oximetry (SpO2).
2. Based on patient presentation and SpO2 readings, apply oxygen via the appropriate device in accordance with local protocols.
3. Auscultate the chest, noting normal or abnormal breath sounds.
4. If indicated and approved by local protocol, administer a breathing treatment or assistance with a bronchodilator inhaler.
5. Consider calling for ALS assistance and do so if you believe the patient may need advanced care beyond your scope of practice.
6. Reassess the patient and repeat vitals every 5–15 minutes as indicated by their severity of distress.
7. Begin preparations for transport if indicated—keep in mind, a focused assessment may be done en route to the hospital.

If the patient has used the inhaler prior to the arrival of EMS, the number of times and amounts administered must be relayed to the medical control, as the patient may have reached or exceeded the maximum dose for that particular medication.

Since most states allow EMTs to administer bronchodilators, you must be familiar with these medications and the methods by which they are administered. Most states will allow, with medical control, the assistance of the EMT in administering the patient's own prescribed inhaler.

Always make sure you follow the **5 Rights** before administering any medication:

1. Is this the right patient?
2. Is this the right medication?
3. Is this the right dosage?
4. Is this the right route of administration?
5. Is this the right time to administer the medication?

Bronchodilator Inhalers

Medications such as Albuterol™, Ventolin™, and Proventil™ are beta-agonist bronchodilators, which quickly and effectively dilate the bronchioles, reducing airway resistance and allowing air to pass more easily and quickly into the alveoli of the lungs.

These medications are only used for patients experiencing dyspnea at the EMT level of care. The patient must already be prescribed an inhaler by their physician, as EMTs do not carry one in their drug box. Thus, if an inhaler is not present with the patient, the only choice of medication at that point is oxygen or CPAP if indicated. ALS may deliver medication through a nebulizer treatment, but the EMT must weigh out the option of traveling to a closer hospital or waiting for ALS to arrive on scene if they had not been called previously.

If medical control gives the order for administration of a handheld metered dose inhaler (MDI), first verify the 5 Rights, and then administer the inhaler as follows:

1. Shake the inhaler vigorously several times and assure that the inhaler is at room temperature.
2. Remove any oxygen adjuncts from the patient, such as a non-rebreather (NRB) mask from the face.
3. Ask the patient to exhale deeply.
4. Ask the patient to place the lips around the mouthpiece of the device and close them, creating a seal.
5. Depress the container as the patient inhales deeply.
6. Ask the patient to hold his breath for as long as possible to allow time for the medication to be absorbed into the tissues of the lungs.
7. Allow the patient to exhale when ready and replace the oxygen adjunct if needed.
8. Reassess the patient.

A patient with a prescribed inhaler will usually have received detailed instructions on its use and may not need all of these details.

Be aware of the possible side effects of these medications, including tachycardia, tremors, and increased anxiety. Be prepared to manage these if and when they occur.

Indications for administration of a prescribed inhaler **must include all of the following criteria**:

- Patient must be exhibiting signs and symptoms of a respiratory emergency.
- Patient's physician must have prescribed the inhaler.
- EMT must have authorization from medical control to administer the medication (unless given service allows administration without medical control permission).

If these conditions are not met, then the use of the inhaler is contraindicated.

Conditions That May Lead to Dyspnea

The EMT must be familiar with the various diseases and conditions that may lead to dyspnea. Common conditions include:

- Asthma
- Chronic obstructive pulmonary disease (COPD), which includes emphysema and chronic bronchitis
- Diabetic ketoacidosis
- Hyperventilation syndrome (can sometimes be psychological)
- Overdose (illicit drugs or otherwise)
- Pneumonia
- Pneumothorax (spontaneous, hemo (blood) or tension based)
- Pulmonary embolism
- Pulmonary edema (many times secondary to congestive heart failure)

Regardless of the reason why the dyspnea is occurring, oxygen saturation must be monitored and corrected as necessary. If respiratory distress begins to go into failure, more aggressive measures must be taken, i.e., OPA/NPA insertion, a BVM, or CPAP.

If BLS medications are indicated for the condition presenting and no contraindications are present, deliver the medication and note whether or not improvement is gained. Be prepared for respiratory or cardiac arrest if it occurs.

Asthma and COPD

Asthma and COPD can both cause similar symptoms: airway constriction, excess mucous production, and shortness of breath when aggravated. However, they are two distinct disease processes.

- **Asthma** is a lifelong inflammatory condition. It is often diagnosed in early childhood but may not present until later in adulthood. There is no cure, but its symptoms can be controlled. Each person is different, and what may trigger one asthmatic may not affect another.
  - For some, asthma is a minor nuisance, and a few puffs of rescue inhaler are all it takes to resolve symptoms.

- For others, asthma can be a major problem that interferes with daily activities and could lead to a life-threatening asthma attack (typically when 911 is activated).
- **Chronic obstructive pulmonary disease** (COPD) is a chronic inflammatory lung disease that causes obstructed airflow from the lungs. It is most commonly seen in patients who have both emphysema and chronic bronchitis.

The **asthma** disease process can be broken down as follows:

- Main problem is that inflammation causes the bronchial airways to narrow, swell, and produce extra mucus.
- Symptoms include coughing, wheezing, and shortness of breath.
- Common "triggers" are pollen, dust, mold, exercise, and even cold weather and humidity.

Treatment of severe asthma attacks will require supplemental high-flow oxygen or possible use of CPAP if no other contraindications exist. ALS treatment includes nebulized breathing medications and possible intubation. The EMT must be able to recognize signs of degrading respiratory efforts, but other factors such as the time waited before a patient called 911 or what medications they have used prior to EMS arrival also matter. The EMT must decide on a course of treatment that not only manages current symptoms but also accounts for possible decompensation if BLS efforts are not successful. This often means an ALS intercept or rapid transport to a hospital for stabilization.

The **COPD** disease process can be broken down as follows:

- Main problem is that chronic inflammation causes narrowing of the bronchial airways and excess mucous production.
- Symptoms include breathing difficulty, cough, mucus production, and wheezing.
- Common "triggers" are cigarette or tobacco smoke, fumes from chemicals and dust, pre-existing asthma or respiratory infection, exercise, hot/cold weather.
- **Treatment** is the same as asthma. Some people with a long-term diagnosis of COPD are very familiar with the use of CPAP during an exacerbation (worsening) of their symptoms and may request that you use that treatment. They may even already know their mask size, which can save you valuable time.

People with COPD often have two additional disease processes occurring at the same time. While they are all separate disease processes, their common symptoms can fan the flames of an already suffering respiratory distress patient. That is why patients are often on multiple medications at the same time—to help manage the dyspnea that can occur.

Put both of these conditions together and it is the recipe for COPD.

- **Emphysema** is a lung disease that destroys the thin walls and elastic fibers of the alveoli. This causes the small airways to collapse when exhaling, which then in turn impairs airflow out of the lungs.
- **Chronic bronchitis** is when the bronchial tubes become inflamed and narrowed, and the lungs then produce more mucus, which increasingly blocks the already narrowed tubes. This leads to a chronic cough, with the patient trying to clear the airways.

Most people with asthma will not develop COPD, and conversely, many people with COPD do not have asthma. However, a few people do have both conditions (called **asthma-COPD overlap syndrome** [ACOS]) and require multiple medications.

Pulmonary Edema and Embolism

Pulmonary is another word associated with the respiratory system. *Pulmonary* specifically refers to the lungs themselves, while *respiratory* refers to the entire system including upper and lower airways.

Pulmonary edema is a condition caused by excess fluid in the lungs. Fluid is pushed from the capillaries into the lungs' air sacs due to the vessels becoming more permeable or "leaky." The collection of fluid in the air sacs makes it hard to breathe (either acutely or over time). If untreated, patients can drown in their own fluids, causing death.

Typically, heart problems such as CHF cause pulmonary edema. However, fluid can accumulate for other reasons, including pneumonia, exposure to toxins or certain medications, trauma to the chest wall, near drowning incidents, and walking at high elevations.

Signs and symptoms vary depending on if it is an acute or chronic condition.

- **Acute**
  - Extreme shortness of breath (SOB) that worsens with movement or lying down
  - Wheezing or gasping for air
  - Cold, clammy skin
  - Anxiety or restlessness
  - Frothy sputum, which may be pink and tinged with blood
  - Rapid, irregular pulse
  - Rales/crackles lung sounds—discontinuous, short bubbling sounds that correspond to the splashing of the fluid in the alveoli during breathing

- **Chronic**
  - More than normal shortness of breath when active
  - Difficulty breathing with exertion or when laying down
  - Possible waking up suddenly with shortness of breath
  - Wheezing, rales, or crackles
  - Swelling of lower extremities
  - Fatigue

Treatment includes monitoring pulse oximetry and delivering appropriate supplemental oxygen either by nasal cannula or non-rebreather mask. Consider ALS and CPAP treatment. Transport to the closest, most appropriate hospital; if the condition is caused by high altitude, a hyperbaric chamber–capable hospital would be a great choice, if available.

Pulmonary embolism is a blockage in one of the pulmonary arteries in the lungs. Most are caused by blood clots that travel to the lungs from deep veins in the legs called a deep vein thrombosis (DVT) or, rarely, from veins in other parts of the body. Some other causes could be air bubbles, fatty marrow clots resulting from a broken bone, or part of a tumor that has broken off and traveled.

Typically, multiple clots are involved, and the parts of lung served by each blocked artery are deprived of blood, causing the tissue to die. This is known as pulmonary infarction. Just like in cardiac infarction, if there is dead tissue this makes it more difficult for your lungs to provide oxygen to the rest of your body.

When conducting your assessment of pulmonary embolism, do the following:

- Ask if the patient has traveled within the last week, particularly the last 48 hours, that involved long periods or sitting
- Ask if the patient has had prolonged bed rest recently (surgery, pregnancy, nursing home patient), as that can increase the risk for pulmonary embolism
- Check to see if the patient is wearing compression stockings; this could help to differentiate between a heart attack, simple dyspnea, or something more complex such as pulmonary embolism
- Get a thorough medication history, as certain birth control medications make women more prone to pulmonary embolism

Signs and symptoms to watch out for are as follows:

- Shortness of breath that comes on suddenly and becomes worse with movement
- Chest pain—often sharp and when breathing in deeply
- Cough that may produce a bloody sputum
- Rapid, irregular heartbeat
- Lightheadedness or dizziness
- Clammy, diaphoretic, or cyanotic skin
- Fever
- Leg pain or swelling, particularly in the calf

Treatment is much the same as any other dyspnea episode. Place supplemental oxygen on with either a nasal cannula or non-rebreather mask. Monitor pulse oximetry and transport to most appropriate hospital. Consider ALS if there is serious deterioration of the patient and if they would be closer than a hospital. Be prepared to provide artificial ventilations if necessary.

Apnea

Apnea is the cessation of breathing. No matter the cause, prompt action must be taken by the EMT, or the heart and rest of the body will cease to function shortly thereafter.

- If a patient is found not breathing, check a pulse immediately in the carotid artery. If there is no pulse after 5–10 seconds, begin CPR starting with chest compressions.
- If you are by yourself, you can use a face mask with a one-way valve to provide breaths after every 30 compressions.

- Ideally, you would use a BVM (bag valve mask), so if one is available, use that to deliver ventilations. If using a BVM, the proper tidal volume is performed (seen with a rise and fall of the chest wall).
  - Once chest rise has occurred, stop squeezing the bag to prevent overinflating the lungs or allowing excess air into the stomach.
  - If there is no chest rise, reposition the head, press down on the mask, and attempt to ventilate again. If after two breaths (or 10 seconds) the chest still does not rise, resume compressions.
- If you feel that it is beginning to become harder to squeeze the BVM bag but you are still getting chest rise, there may be something internally occurring such as a tension pneumothorax or an airway obstruction. Communicate with your partner that it is becoming more difficult; if ALS has not already been contacted, the decision to do so or begin to transport emergently must be made here.
- If you suspect an obstruction is the cause of the apnea, open the mouth and attempt to locate the object. If it cannot be seen, do NOT perform a blind finger sweep per AHA standards. If chest compressions are being performed, the pressure built up from doing so within the chest cavity may be enough to force the object out of the airway. Have the person completing the ventilations do periodic airway checks to see if the object appears. If it does not, ALS or the hospital has tools that can be used to visualize and remove the object.
- If you suspect a medical reason is the cause of the apnea and the patient still has a pulse (as with drug overdose or anaphylaxis), you may need to administer medication such as naloxone or epinephrine. That could prompt the patient to begin breathing on their own.

No matter the cause of the apnea, it is up to the EMT to correct the situation as soon as possible before complete death happens.

Airway Management

Artificial Ventilation

In the event of poor or absent respirations, artificial ventilation of the patient may be required. This is accomplished by forcing air into the lungs, utilizing a technique known as positive pressure ventilation (PPV).

There are multiple ways to perform PPV: mouth-to-mask, bag-valve mask, oxygen-demand valve, and CPAP.

Mouth-to-Mask

Mouth-to-mask (or pocket mask) ventilation is used when there is no other EMS equipment available, to sustain a patient's oxygen-saturation level until more effective ventilation can be achieved. It is commonly used in EMS.

The mouth-to-mask is available as an individual package or as a set with a bag-valve mask. If packaged individually, it should come with a one-way valve to help protect the rescuer.

To provide effective breaths mouth to mask, it is imperative that the mask be tightly sealed to the patient's face.

- Use an E-C clamp where the thumb and index finger hold the mask down over the nose and mouth of the patient, forming a C.
- The other three fingers of your hand should grasp the patient's mandible, forming an E.

Then, tilt the head back using the other hand (or use the jaw-thrust maneuver if trauma is suspected).

- If the person has a pulse and requires only rescue breaths, give one breath every 5–6 seconds.
- If the person is pulseless and not breathing adequately on her own, do CPR in conjunction with breaths.
  - Use a 30:2 rhythm, i.e., 30 compressions and two breaths.
  - Deliver each breath over 1 second, with each breath producing visible chest rise.

Bag-Valve Mask

Bag-valve mask (BVM) ventilation provides a higher concentration of oxygen than exhaled air and lessens the contact with biological hazards for both the patient and the EMT. A tight seal is also imperative between the mask and the face.

- Use a one-handed "C" technique, as described for the pocket mask.
- Connect the bag to the opening at the top of the mask, if this has not already been done.
- Use the other hand to squeeze the bag and push air into the patient.
  - Be careful to squeeze the bag only until you see chest rise, and then stop.
  - That will reduce the chances of barotrauma, overinflation of the lungs, or air entering into the stomach.
- The most efficient way to use a BVM is to use the two-person technique: one person maintains a mask seal, while the second person ventilates with the bag.

The BVM also comes with an oxygen inlet port, which allows the patient to be ventilated with 100% oxygen. An experienced EMT can feel in the resistance of the bag the efficiency of the ventilation effort, as well as noting the patient's chest rise and the exhalation of air after inspiration.

If the bag becomes increasingly harder to squeeze, reassess the airway, as a number of things could be wrong.

- Check the mask seal to make sure it is still intact with the face.
- Check the airway to make sure it is not obstructed by fluids or objects. Suction if necessary.
- Check to see if the airway is positioned properly and readjust if needed.

- Consider things such as a tension pneumothorax.
- If the patient is intubated by an ALS provider, have that person check the position of the tube placement. Communicate that you are feeling resistance and it is becoming harder to squeeze the BVM.

Oxygen-Demand Valve

The oxygen-powered ventilation device provides the same type of ventilation but with less physical exertion, as it is does not require one to squeeze a bag to inflate the lungs. This method uses a demand valve that is controlled by respiration rate, allowing increased oxygen flow in response to increased demand. However, the mask must be sealed on the face as with both the pocket mask and the BVM.

Many EMS services have discontinued the oxygen-powered device, as many EMTs feel that the BVM gives better control of artificial ventilation and that with an oxygen hookup the amount of oxygen delivered with either device is 100%.

With the increase in communicable diseases that can be spread by intimate contact, mouth-to-mouth resuscitation is now used less and less. Practically speaking, the only time it is used today is when the EMT is reasonably certain that there is no risk of contamination.

Continuous Positive Airway Pressure (CPAP)

Airway collapse can result from many conditions, and one of the tools now available to many EMTs (state-dependent) is the use of CPAP.

Via a specialized face mask, CPAP forces a small amount of air pressure through the bronchioles and into the alveoli, causing them to reopen. The pressure created by CPAP is held constant throughout the breathing cycle. During inspiration, the patient may feel a small amount of pressure (versus a regular breath), and during exhalation may feel the same thing.

For patients using a CPAP for the first time, it can be a very strange feeling—one that may require convincing to accept. Moreover, the patient may not be thinking clearly (often due to hypoxia), and even though you know that CPAP will help alleviate the breathing, it might feel suffocating to the patient. This is when a good patient rapport and patience can go a long way in compliance.

In conditions that cause excess fluid in the lungs, such as heart failure, drowning, and pulmonary edema, the gas exchange between carbon dioxide and oxygen occurs within the lungs' alveoli. Each alveoli has a liquid called **surfactant**, which reduces water surface tension within the pleural space and keeps the alveolus open. If the fluid balance is disturbed, this will cause the alveoli to collapse, a condition called **atelectasis**. That in turn will compromise the gas exchange process, and the patient will start to experience respiratory distress.

CPAP may also be indicated for several other conditions where the gas exchange process is disrupted:

- Bronchoconstriction, e.g., asthma and COPD in moderate to severe distress
- Toxic gases, e.g., chemicals or smoke inhalation that cause bronchoconstriction and swelling
- Flail chest: insufficient chest rise as a result of broken ribs and pain (CPAP can support proper tidal volumes)
- Lung infections, e.g., pneumonia and any other infection that occurs within the lungs

A main concern with CPAP is that it can lower blood pressure. (As pressure increases inside the lungs, the pressure on the heart chambers and great vessels also increases, thus causing cardiac output to drop.) Contraindications for CPAP use are as follows:

- Reduced level of consciousness or unconsciousness
- Inability to protect their own airway
- Cardiac or respiratory arrest
- Facial trauma that would prevent a good mask seal (broken bones, burns, etc.)
- Copious secretions in the mouth
- Severe nausea with vomiting

Oxygen-Delivery Systems

Oxygen

Oxygen is the most widely used drug by EMS and is indicated in almost all protocols for difficulty breathing, as well as many other conditions such as chest pain. Consequently, it is carried aboard all EMS vehicles and used routinely by EMTs.

- The **onboard** system is stored in an "M" cylinder, which contains 3,000 liters of oxygen.
- The **portable** system (carried to a patient) is stored in a smaller "D" or "E" cylinder, each of which carries 350 and 625 liters of oxygen, respectively.
  - Cylinders are filled to a maximum pressure of 2,000 pounds per square inch and must be handled with great care.

- If heated, a full cylinder may rupture and cause an explosion that can easily kill a bystander.

- Keep at least one hand on the cylinder at all times, as it may also become a projectile if dropped at a certain angle.

To be used for EMS purposes, the pressure must be reduced by a pressure regulator, which is attached to the valve of the tank. This regulator can then be adjusted to provide the proper flow to the patient in liters per minute (lpm).

Masks

Oxygen is delivered to the patient through a mask that fits over the nose and mouth or through a prong that fits into the nostrils. Masks come in different styles, as per the percentage of oxygen required.

- A **full non-rebreather mask (NRB)** at a flow rate of 10–15 liters/minute delivers almost 100% oxygen.
- A **simple face mask** at a flow rate of 6–10 liters/minute delivers 40–60% oxygen.
- A **nasal cannula (NC)** at a flow rate of 2–6 liters/minute delivers 20–40% oxygen.
- A **Venturi mask** is an adjustable type of mask with a flow rate from 2–15 liters/minute and delivers 24–60% oxygen depending on which of the color-coded valves is chosen.

The choice of device is predicated on the patient's degree of **hypoxia** (low oxygen). A pulse oximeter is very useful for this task. A patient who presents with cyanosis requires more oxygen than one who presents with normal skin color and an inability to catch his breath.

- A patient who complains of difficulty breathing yet has normal color and pulse oximeter reading in the high 90s may be given an NC.
- A pale patient with saturation below 90% probably needs a higher concentration device, such as an NRB.

Treat the patient, not the equipment. Look at the overall patient presentation to determine the proper treatment sequence.

- A potential carbon dioxide victim may produce a false reading of 100% SpO_2 if you do not have a dual-reader for both oxygen and carbon dioxide.
- Be careful in cases of stroke and myocardial infarction. Studies have shown that 100% oxygen rates may be harming patients; instead, the ideal pulse oximeter reading is 92–98% with a flow rate 2–4 liters/min.

TEST YOURSELF 5.2

What type of oxygen would you provide this patient?

You respond to your local nursing home facility for a patient who has fallen. Upon arrival, you find an 87-year-old male laying on the floor next to his bed and a staff member who hands you paperwork. The staff member states that she doesn't know what happened as she "just came on shift and when doing her rounds, found him on the floor like this and was afraid to move him." The patient is normally on 2 lpm of oxygen with a nasal cannula (which is not on his face at this time). Vital signs are BP 118/58 mm Hg, pulse 82, respiratory rate 14, and pulse oximetry 93%. He is not in any obvious respiratory distress.

Do you give this patient oxygen? If yes, what delivery device and at how many liters would you provide?

Practice Set

1. You are a BLS unit and are dispatched to a local nursing home for a patient with difficulty breathing. Upon entering the patient's room, you find two nurses standing over a 70-year-old male lying supine in bed. His breathing is distressed and he is using his accessory muscles to breathe. The nurses explain that they "found him this way" during their routine check. His respiratory rate is 34 and shallow, his oxygen saturation is 78%, and he is pale. You are wearing universal precautions, and there is no indication of any scene safety issues. What would be your next move?

    A. Place the patient on 12 liters per minute oxygen via a non-rebreather mask

    B. Open the patient's airway using a head-tilt, chin-lift

    C. Ventilate the patient with a bag-valve mask

    D. Request an Advanced Life Support intercept

2. You are dispatched to a residence for a child not breathing. The scene is safe, and you are wearing gloves. Entering the living room, you see a 4-year-old child lying on his back and his mother nearby screaming, "My baby, my baby!" You approach the child and take stabilization of the head and look, listen, and feel for air exchange; none is noted. You perform a modified jaw thrust and again look, listen, and feel, and air exchange is still negative. You instruct your partner to attempt to ventilate, and she advises you that there appears to be an obstruction. You reposition the airway, and she tries again with no success. What is your next instruction?

    A. Call 911

    B. Examine the airway

    C. Perform a blind finger sweep to feel for an object

    D. Roll the patient over and perform five back blows

3. When you examine the airway, you see a small toy truck about 2 inches long in the back of oropharynx. What suction device would you tell your partner to use to remove it?

    A. A 14-gauge soft-tip French catheter

    B. Rigid-tip Yankauer catheter

    C. Untipped suction hose

    D. Her fingers

4. Which of the following are the correct landmarks for sizing a nasopharyngeal airway?

   A. Tip of ear to tip of nose

   B. Tip of ear to corner of mouth

   C. Corner of mouth to tip of nose

   D. Corner of mouth to tip of ear

5. Which of the following is a contraindication for use of a nasopharyngeal airway?

   A. Apnea

   B. Seizure

   C. Facial trauma

   D. Pulse oximetry saturation reading less than 90%

6. Which of the following should be used to lubricate a nasopharyngeal airway?

   A. Petroleum jelly

   B. Olive oil

   C. Water-soluble lubricant

   D. Your saliva

7. You respond to a residence for a call for difficulty breathing. In the bedroom is a 40-year-old female sitting up in bed in severe respiratory distress. She is pale, and you note that her neck muscles are protruded. She is breathing at a rate of 30. The patient tries to say, "Can't breathe," but is barely able to speak. Her pulse oximetry is 72% on room air. Her husband explains that she has a history of emphysema, for which she takes medication. She is not on supplemental oxygen. She has no other pertinent history and no allergies. Auscultation of her chest, sides, and back reveal the presence of rhonchi in all fields. Which of the following is the most appropriate first treatment?

   A. Administer two puffs of her Albuterol inhaler

   B. Administer liquid albuterol through a nebulizer mask

   C. Administer oxygen via nasal cannula at 6 liters per minute

   D. Administer oxygen via non-rebreather mask at 15 liters per minute

8. You are transporting the patient in question 7 to the emergency department. Her pulse oximetry has risen to 92% with supplemental oxygen, and her respiratory rate is now down to 20 breaths per minute. Suddenly she becomes unconscious, and you notice she has stopped breathing. You open her airway and she still does not breathe spontaneously and has no gag reflex, and you do not see any secretions. What devices, in the correct order, would you utilize next?

   A. CPAP, OPA, NPA, suction

   B. Suction, NPA, BVM

   C. OPA, BVM

   D. BVM, NPA, OPA

9. You respond to a residence for a call for difficulty breathing. You enter the bedroom of a 60-year-old female, seated with her shoulders hunched forward in respiratory distress. Her pulse oximetry is 78%, her respiratory rate is 30, and she is pale and diaphoretic. Auscultation of the lungs reveals a crackling-type sound in the posterior bases. This type of sound is referred to as which of the following?

   A. Rales

   B. Rhonchi

   C. Stridor

   D. Wheezing

10. In the scenario in question 9, which of the following is the most correct immediate intervention?

   A. Lie the patient down and perform an airway maneuver

   B. Request an ALS intercept

   C. Administer oxygen 6 liters per minute via nasal cannula

   D. Administer oxygen 15 liters per minute via non-rebreather mask

11. While attempting to ventilate a patient who has stopped breathing while en route to the hospital, you insert an OPA and place a BVM over the patient's mouth and nose and squeeze the bag. You note that there is not much resistance and that the patient's chest does not rise. Which of the following is the most likely cause of this failure?

   A. Inadequate oxygen supply

   B. Equipment failure

   C. Failure to pre-oxygenate the patient

   D. Failure to seal the mask against the patient's face

12. Which of the following best describes the method for inserting an oropharyngeal airway (OPA)?

   A. Depress the tongue and slide the OPA in

   B. Rotate the OPA 180 degrees and insert, twisting it 180 degrees once it passes the tongue

   C. Rotate the OPA 180 degrees and insert it into the airway

   D. Depress the tongue and insert the OPA, rotating it 360 degrees in the airway

13. While conducting your truck check at the beginning of your shift, you notice that the onboard oxygen system tank has no pressure left. What size tank should you replace it with?

   A. D

   B. E

   C. M

   D. X

Answers and Explanations

1. B

After ensuring that the scene is safe and you are wearing universal precautions, your next step in the medical scenario is *always* to ensure that your patient has a patent airway. The other answer choices are all treatments you may wish to consider after that time.

2. B

The patient may have aspirated a foreign object, causing the airway blockage. (A) is not correct because you *are* 911, although you may want additional help or an ALS intercept. (D) is a potential option once you have completed step (B) first. The blind finger sweep (C) has been removed from AHA standards.

3. D

A blockage of this type can be removed by grasping it with two fingers and removing it from the airway. (A), (B), and (C) are all suction devices designed for fluids, which will probably be ineffective in removing an object as large as this.

4. A

The correct answer is (A). (B) and (D) are the correct answers for an oropharyngeal airway, and (C) is not used for any airway device.

5. C

Facial trauma contraindicates use of the nasopharyngeal airway due to the possibility of an opening into the cranium that would allow the device to penetrate into that compartment and complicate the fracture. Apnea (A) is the absence of breathing, which would indicate use of an airway adjunct to assist with ventilations. Seizure (B) often indicates the use of an NPA, versus an OPA, due to teeth clenching, and pulse oximetry saturation <90% (D) is an indication that oxygen perfusion is needed.

6. C

Petroleum jelly (A) will break down the material of the NPA. Olive oil (B) will not lubricate sufficiently, and its liquidity may cause choking. Your saliva (D) is completely unacceptable, unsanitary, and unsterile. Use a water-soluble lubricant.

7. D

(A) is a possible treatment but not for the level of distress she is currently experiencing, and (B) is a treatment that is typically only an ALS skill. The key to the remaining answer choices is in the pulse oximetry reading of 72%, which indicates severe hypoxia. A rate of 6 liters per minute (C) will help raise her oxygen saturation, but not as quickly as 15 liters per minute. Remember that a nasal cannula only delivers a maximum of 40% oxygen, while a non-rebreather will deliver almost 100%.

8. C

You would use OPA and then BVM, choice (C). First, provide artificial ventilation to the patient. Once you have manually opened the airway, use an OPA to assist in maintaining the airway, and ventilate with a BVM using supplemental oxygen. There is no indication here for the use of suction (B) or an NPA (A).

9. A

Rales are a fine crackling sound caused by fluid in the alveoli and are usually an indication of pulmonary edema, most often caused by congestive heart failure. Rhonchi are snoring-type sounds, stridor is a high-pitched sound coming from the upper airway, and wheezing is a lower pitched sound coming from the bronchi being constricted.

10. D

A conscious patient with pulmonary edema will be unable to breathe if you try to lay her down in a supine position, and she will resist your efforts to do so. Pulmonary edema can be treated with ALS drugs, but your patient's immediate need is oxygen perfusion, which you can accomplish with supplemental oxygen. (C) is too low of an oxygen flow for this particular patient presentation, while (D) would provide better and faster relief.

11. D

Lack of resistance when squeezing the bag means that the air is going somewhere else. Equipment failure, such as a leak in the bag or mask, is a possibility, but not likely. The percentages of oxygen and pre-oxygenation, while important to the patient's condition, have nothing to do with the physical ventilation of the lungs.

12. B

The oropharyngeal airway should be rotated 180 degrees from the anatomical position and inserted into the mouth. Once the airway passes the tongue, it should be rotated 180 degrees back to the anatomical position.

13. C

D and E cylinders are for portable use, and there is no such thing as an X tank for emergency medical oxygen.

CHAPTER 6

Medical Emergencies

Topics Discussed

- **Pharmacology**
- **Cardiovascular Emergencies**
- **Altered Mental Status, Strokes, and TIAs**
- **Shock and Sepsis**
- **Diabetes, Seizures, and Allergic Reaction Emergencies**
- **Poisoning, Overdose, and Environmental Emergencies**
- **Behavioral Emergencies**
- **Obstetric and Gynecological Emergencies**

In the practice of prehospital emergency medicine, the EMT will come across many varied medical emergencies involving one or more body systems. The EMT will also be responsible for being able to recognize when and how to administer various medications or when to call for ALS if a call goes beyond their scope of practice.

If you notice that respiratory emergencies are not mentioned in this chapter, please refer back to chapter 5 for a more in-depth look at airway and related emergencies.

Pharmacology

An EMT may be instructed to administer medication to a patient in the field. Therefore, it is important to understand what these medications are, how they work, for what medical conditions they are administered (indications), and under which circumstances they should not be administered (contraindications).

The EMT must always be guided by the local protocols as to drug administration, since these protocols vary widely by location.

According to the latest National EMS Scope of Practice Model, there are nine medications that an EMT can administer in the field. The seven most common ones follow:

Table 6.1 *Most Common Medications That EMTs Can Deliver*

Medication	Dosage	Route
Oxygen	1–25 liters per minute (lpm) depending on route and oxygen regulator used* *Many regulators range only from 2–15 lpm and are more familiar to the EMT	• Nasal cannula (NC): 2–6 lpm • Non-rebreather (NRB): 10–25 lpm • BVM: 2–15 lpm • Venturi may be adjusted individually to patient • CPAP: typically preset to 10 lpm start, but follow directions or training by your service
Oral glucose	10–50 grams	• Buccal route preferably • Typically given in a pre-dosed (10–15 g) tube that must be opened and delivered to a conscious patient who is able to protect her own airway
Epinephrine	Adults: 0.3 mg Pediatrics: 0.15 mg	• Given intramuscular (IM) in outer lateral thigh • Typically given via auto-injector but some states may allow EMTs to draw from a vial using a syringe
Aspirin (ASA)	Tablets, available in 325 mg or 81 mg	• Orally and chewed (must be non-enteric coated tablets) • If using 325 mg: give 1 tablet • If using 81 mg: give 4 tablets
Opioid antagonists (Naloxone/Narcan)	Available in 2 mg/mL or 0.4 mg/mL	• Intranasal (IN): 2 mg/mL with 1 mL delivered per nostril in a pre-filled syringe • Intramuscular (IM): 0.4 mg/mL typically drawn up from a 1 mL vial (allowed only in some states)
Bronchodilators (e.g., albuterol, ventolin, ipratropium)	Dosage depends on patient's prescription	• Most typically encountered in metered dose-inhalers (MDIs) • Typically given 1–2 puffs per administration (read prescription) • Patient may use a "spacer," a specialized tube that allows for aerosolized particles to remain airborne longer (popular in pediatric or geriatric populations)
Nitroglycerin (Nitro)	0.4 mg or 1/150th grain	• Oral dissolving tablet: place under tongue and let melt; do not chew, crush, or swallow • Spray: lift tongue and deliver sublingually 1 spray at a time • Paste: (allowed only in some states)

Familiarize yourself with the more common prescription medications, as they can be clues to potential problems. This is especially helpful for situations where a patient is found alone and unresponsive. By locating a patient's prescription (in a bag, etc.), you can get an idea of the type of medical condition you are dealing with, either in an acute form or chronic basis.

Antidotes for chemical/hazardous materials exposure, **activated charcoal**, and **glucagon** are also available at the BLS level nationally; however, not all states allow their administration by the EMT and thus may not be tested on the exam. All EMTs should know which medications are allowed within their scope of practice.

Medications may be administered to the patient in a variety of ways.

Table 6.2 *Medication Routes*

Route	Shorthand Written Form	How Given	Forms Medications May Come In
Injection	Intramuscular (IM) or subcutaneous (Sub-Q)	• For IM, insert needle catheter at 90° angle into a muscle such as buttocks or deltoid muscle • For sub-Q, inject needle catheter into the layer between skin and muscle, into the fatty tissue	• Liquid in pre-filled syringes, which may be manual or auto-injectors
Inhalation/ Aerosolized (nebulizer administration by EMT allowed only in some states)	INH	Depress the prescribed inhaler/canister, and airborne droplets will be released into the patient's mouth and airway	• Suspensions • Gases • Liquids • Aerosols
Oral	PO	Place medication into the mouth of the patient; some medications are meant to be swallowed, while others are meant to melt onto the tongue	• Tablets • Capsules
Buccal	BUC	Place medication inside the cheek, between the teeth and cheek tissue	• Gels • Liquids
Sublingual	SL	Place medication underneath the patient's tongue	• Tablets • Sprays
Rectal (allowed by EMT only in some states)	REC	Place medication in the rectum	• Suppositories • Gels

Accredited programs are responsible for teaching the national curriculum, not just the state protocols in which the course is located. This is why the EMT may see medication questions on the NREMT exam that may not apply to their particular state allowances.

Medication Rights

Medication errors harm an estimated 1.5 million people per year, and as health care providers, EMTs are included as one of the causes for this alarming statistic.

Many EMS systems allow the EMT to administer medication that is already prescribed for a particular patient, e.g., asthma medication administered by metered dose inhaler such as albuterol, metaproterenol, and ipratropium; nitroglycerin for angina; and epinephrine for anaphylaxis.

When administering medication, the EMT must know the "medication rights" of drug therapy. Many programs still teach the 5 Rights, but there are additional rights that should also be kept in mind for the practitioner. In the list below, these additional rights are indicated with an asterisk (*). They are:

- Is this the right medication?
- Is this the right patient? (especially important for prescriptions)
- Is this the right route of administration?
- Is this the right dosage?
- Is this the right date? (expiration date has not passed)
- *Is this the right time to take the medication? (scheduled doses such as insulin or overdose errors)
- *Is this the right response to the medication? (allergic reactions or adverse reactions)
- *Is this right reason for the medication? (e.g., glucose auto-injector instead of an epinephrine auto-injector)

When medication is administered, note the date and time and document them in your run report. Following the drug administration, reassess the patient to see if there are any changes in condition, including vital signs.

Cardiovascular Emergencies

One of the most common emergency calls is for chest pain. Chest pain can be caused by many things, including cardiovascular issues, musculoskeletal issues, or even cardiac arrest. It is up to the EMT, along with good assessment skills, to be able to differentiate the various causes and administer the proper treatment.

Heart issues can be broken down into three categories:

- Is it an electrical problem?
- Is it a circulatory problem?
- Is it a structural problem?

Electrical Problems

Electrical problems stem from the heart's electrical pathways not functioning correctly or at all. Some terms to know when speaking about electrical issues are as follows:

- **Arrhythmia/dysrhythmia**: irregular rate or rhythm
- **Tachycardia**: fast heart rate
- **Bradycardia**: slow heart rate
- **Asystole**: no electrical impulses produced ("flatline")
- **Fibrillation** (atrial or ventricular): the heart is "shaking" but there is no squeezing of the blood into other parts of the heart

It is not within the National Scope of Practice for EMTs to know all of the heart rhythms or interpret them on an EKG. However, you should be able to recognize that an arrhythmia/dysrhythmia will result in various medical conditions that range from chronic diseases (e.g., atrial fibrillation) to sudden cardiac arrest (SCA). Ventricular fibrillation is considered a lethal rhythm.

Circulatory Problems

Circulatory problems deal with issues that arise from the vessels supplying or leaving the heart or from the fluid that flows within the heart itself.

Table 6.3 *Common Circulatory Problems*

Circulatory Problem	Issues It Can Cause
Hypertension (HTN)	• Develops when steady pressure on vessel walls weakens them over time • If the vessel is weaker, it becomes more susceptible to deposit buildup which may eventually break off and travel to the heart or brain; result can be myocardial infarction (heart attack) or stroke • Vessel failure can happen as well, with aneurysms occurring
Coronary Artery Disease (CAD)	• Develops when major blood vessels that supply the heart (the coronary arteries) become damaged or diseased • Plaque deposits and inflammation occur • Vessels narrow, not allowing adequate blood flow and leading to angina pain, shortness of breath, or complete blockage leading to myocardial infarction

(Continued)

Table 6.3 *Common Circulatory Problems (Continued)*

Circulatory Problem	Issues It Can Cause
Arteriosclerosis/ Atherosclerosis (called "hardening of the arteries")	• Develops when blood flow is restricted, making the arterial walls hard and stiff (normally, they are soft and flexible); causes various symptoms depending on the artery that has been affected • Result is a buildup of plaques in the arteries • Lifestyle changes may reverse or relieve symptoms (smoking cessation, weight loss, healthier diet)
Angina or Angina Pectoris	• Type of chest pain that develops from reduced blood flow to the heart • Typically unexpected, so be sure to ask OPQRST questions thoroughly • **Stable angina** goes away with medication or rest • **Unstable angina** does not typically go away with rest or medication and may signal that a heart attack is about to occur
Myocardial Infarction (MI)	• Develops when plaque buildup has completely occluded one of the heart's vessels; causes the surrounding heart tissue to become hypoxic and toxins to build up • If not treated quickly, may result in cardiac arrest; if caught in time, may require stents to keep arteries open for long term
Hypoperfusion Syndrome (Shock)	• Circulation is inadequate to the various organs of the body • May be caused by low fluid volume (hypovolemia) or inadequate pumping of the heart (such as congestive heart failure [CHF]) • Can lead to electrical problems and arrythmias • Look for traumatic causes vs. medical causes and treat accordingly
Acute Coronary Syndrome (ACS)	• Describes a range of conditions associated with sudden, reduced blood flow to the heart • If ACS does not result in an MI, it will typically alter the blood flow temporarily or permanently, which may result in creating unstable angina • Often places patient at higher risk for stroke and heart attack in the future

Structural Problems

Structural problems stem from damage to the heart itself. This can be a result of a traumatic injury or issues such as:

- **Congestive heart failure (CHF)**, when the left or right ventricle is weakened to the point that it no longer has the strength to pump blood properly to the lungs or the body
  - Common causes: diabetes, HTN, and CAD
  - Signs and symptoms: fluid buildup in the lungs, extremity edema (swelling), tiredness, and shortness of breath
- **Cardiac tamponade**, an acute condition where blood or fluids fill the pericardial sac that surrounds the heart itself; places extreme pressure on the heart and prevents the heart's ventricles from expanding fully (if not released, can prevent the heart from beating entirely)

- Classic symptoms (Beck's triad): hypotension, muffled heart sounds, and jugular vein distention (JVD)
- Other symptoms: restlessness, anxiety, clammy extremities, and tachycardia
- **Pericardial effusion**, similar to cardiac tamponade but with a slower buildup of fluids

Treatment (Emergency Care)

While EMTs are not able to definitively diagnose and treat the various cardiac conditions above, they must be able to differentiate between the various possibilities in the field so that they can have a working diagnosis (and eventual treatment).

If you come upon a cardiac-compromised patient, you must be alert that this is an ALS situation and requires either an intercept or rapid transport to an emergency department. With the patient's best interests in mind, you must make a decision about which of these two options to execute, based upon the time each will require. The longer that definitive treatment (either medical or surgical) is delayed, the more there can be damage to the heart tissue.

Emergency care of the suspected cardiac compromise falls into two categories:

- **No pulse?** Move on to possible defibrillation with an AED and CPR.
- **Pulse present?** Move on to the initial assessment, focused history, and physical exam.

Obtain baseline vital signs, including pulse oximetry, and apply oxygen as appropriate. Also consider giving cardiac medications if indicated.

The OPQRST series of questions is important in the proper assessment of chest pain and will be communicated to the emergency department so that personnel there may properly triage the patient. Especially important is the description of the quality of the pain and whether it is stationary or radiating. Remember that time is tissue in a heart attack (myocardial infarction). If the EMT has performed an adequate focused exam and relays a complete picture to the triage nurse, then time is saved at the triage desk, and the patient is processed quickly to a more definitive level of care that may minimize the damage to the patient's heart.

Medication

Current studies have shown that aspirin, taken daily as a prophylactic or given at the onset of chest pain, dramatically improves a patient's chances of survival. Consequently, many local protocols now call for the EMT to administer aspirin to chest-pain patients, providing they have not already taken one.

Many times, the patient has already had a prior episode and may have been prescribed nitroglycerin (NTG) tablets or spray to treat sudden onset chest pain. If your local protocol allows you to administer NTG or assist the patient in administering it, check with your medical control and follow all directions.

Be sure to ask if the patient has taken any erectile dysfunction medication (this includes females) in the last 24–48 hours, as that could cause an unsafe drop in blood pressure when given with NTG.

NTG is a powerful vasodilator that is placed sublingually and is rapidly absorbed, causing the arteries to dilate.

Side effects may include a drop in blood pressure and headache. If the chest pain is alleviated with NTG, then the physician may suspect that the cause of the chest pain is not myocardial infarction, but instead it may be angina.

Be sure that the patient's systolic blood pressure is higher than 100 mm Hg when giving NTG, since a drop in blood pressure may result in hypotension that can lead to hypoxia. Continue retaking the blood pressure once you have administered NTG to monitor the effect of the drug.

CPR and Automated External Defibrillators (AED)

While not every chest-pain patient is going to lapse into cardiac arrest, it can and does happen. Continued assessment is important in these cases. If the patient does suddenly go into cardiac arrest, you must be prepared to respond immediately.

- Always travel with the devices you would need to do CPR: the AED (automated external defibrillator), a bag-valve mask, OPAs, and suctioning equipment.
  - An AED is a computer-driven device that analyzes a patient's cardiac rhythm and determines whether a countershock is advised. The purpose of this countershock is to re-establish a perfusing rhythm.
  - Current research indicates that if the patient's heart is in ventricular tachycardia or ventricular fibrillation, a shock delivered as soon as possible after the condition occurs could convert the irregular rhythm to a rhythm that would once again generate a pulse.
  - An exception is if the patient is in an asystole rhythm, or pulseless electrical activity (PEA), which will cause the AED to state "no shock advised, continue CPR if necessary." This type of heart rhythm will respond only to high-quality CPR and cardiac medication administered by ALS providers or hospital personnel. Depending on how long the patient is in this rhythm, they may never recover and become deceased, despite the EMT's best efforts.

The AED does not take the place of CPR, but is an adjunct to it. As of this printing, the AHA suggests the following sequence for an adult patient:

Table 6.4 *How to Use an AED (Adults Only)*

Step Number	Direction
1	Determine if the scene is safe and that appropriate infection control precautions are in place.
2	If CPR in progress, stop it and verify that the patient has no pulse and is not breathing.
3	Have your partner continue CPR while you prepare and attach the AED pads in the correct placement as indicated by the pictures. Listen and follow the prompts as indicated. Do not touch the patient during the analyze cycle.
4	If the AED states "shock advised," continue with chest compressions while the AED charges. When the light or sound is made alerting that the machine is charged, ALL personnel (including whomever is on airway) must stand clear while the shock button is depressed. Immediately resume compressions.
5	If the AED indicates "no shock advised, begin CPR if necessary," perform a pulse and breathing check. If these are absent, immediately resume chest compressions.
6	Use the following guidelines for chest compressions: • Perform at a rate of 100–120/minute using 2 hands • Compress at least 2–2.4 inches (5–6 cm) in depth • Keep your elbows and arms locked with shoulder located directly over the patient's body
7	Continue providing compressions and breaths in a 30:2 ratio until either ALS arrives or you have made the decision to rapidly transport to avoid delay on scene.
8	If the AED has restored the pulse, check the patient continually for a pulse. If the pulse disappears, repeat the CPR/AED steps.

Some EMS systems are performing what is called **cardiocerebral resuscitation**, or CCR. This differs from CPR in that for the first 5–10 minutes after cardiac arrest, a rescuer does not breathe for the patient at all. Instead, the focus shifts to performing continuous chest compressions at a rate of 100–120/min. This has shown positive results in resuscitation in some studies, but as always the EMT must follow the local protocols.

Discontinuing CPR and Biological Death

Sometimes, despite the EMT's best efforts, a patient will not obtain a return of spontaneous circulation (ROSC), where a pulse comes back and the person recovers from cardiac arrest.

Stop doing CPR under the following situations:

- Patient obtains and maintains ROSC
- Verified and legal DNR (do not resuscitate) order has been produced
- Physician has ordered discontinuation of CPR
- Signs of obvious biological death are present

    - Decapitation of the head
    - Rigor mortis/rigidity of body

- Lividity (blue bruise-like coloring) in the trunk of body or extremities
- Decomposition of the entire body
- Burned beyond recognition with no pulse or breathing present

Certain EMS systems allow for their providers to initiate a "field termination" after meeting criteria laid out by their protocols, while other systems require a physician to order cessation of efforts done.

Regarding the **do not resuscitate (DNR) order**, each state has its own rules on what makes one valid or not. Typically, they all follow some general rules:

- A physician must physically sign the paper.
- The patient's full legal name must be included.
- It must be dated; some papers will have expiration dates to re-discuss options.

Some states may also require the following:

- DNR must be on a specific form (which may or may not be colored)
- Paper must be produced within 2 minutes before resuscitation efforts commence
- Some may only withhold compressions, but will allow artificial ventilation efforts
- Provide a photograph of the patient, for additional verification against the name on the form

As always, be familiar with your system's protocols and standards.

Altered Mental Status and Stroke

Altered Mental Status

Altered mental status (AMS), also called altered level of consciousness (ALOC), is an umbrella term for any type of behavior that is abnormal from the patient's baseline normal mental function. It can be caused by many things, from cerebral hemorrhage to trauma, drug overdose, and many disease processes.

The overall goal for the EMT is to find out the root cause of the AMS and try to fix the presenting symptoms. The only way to get to this route cause is to do a proper and thorough assessment.

AMS patients are usually not alert and oriented, thus they are unable to provide the EMT with very reliable information. If they are somewhat conscious, AMS makes it difficult to communicate, which could equate to the patient struggling to describe the signs or symptoms. They may even give vague answers because they only know that "something" is wrong but are unable to pinpoint exactly what that "something" is.

Any bystanders available, especially those who know the patient, can provide very useful information:

- Verification that the information given by the patient is correct
- Attestation of the patient's normal baseline mental status
- Details that can "fill in the blanks" about the situation

Keep in mind that AMS may be just one of multiple problems going on at once and that doing a thorough assessment can catch issues that may otherwise be dismissed. This is especially true of repeat 911 callers, where EMS providers may shortcut an assessment due to "they were fine the last few times we came." Don't let a distracting injury or illness deter you from finding out why the injury/illness occurred in the first place.

- Suppose you give a presumed hypoglycemic patient oral glucose in the proper dosage, but she does not respond as you would expect (which would be to wake up and become alert and oriented). Now suppose you do a complete neurological check, noting left arm drift. Now you suspect a stroke in addition to the hypoglycemic event.

- Suppose you are dispatched to a fall victim who has an open femur fracture. You may be tempted to deal with just the injury and not find out that the fall was caused by a stroke whose symptoms came on suddenly.

A helpful mnemonic to remember the potential causes of AMS is **AEIOU-TIPS**:

- **A**: alcohol
- **E**: epilepsy *(seizures)*
- **I**: insulin *(diabetic issues?)*
- **O**: overdose *(too much of a drug?)*
- **U**: underdose/uremia *(too little or no dose of a drug? or toxins buildup from renal disease?)*
- **T**: toxins/trauma/temperature
- **I**: infection *(sepsis? pneumonia? urinary tract infection?)*
- **P**: psychosis/poisoning *(carbon monoxide? pesticides?)*
- **S**: stroke

Every patient should receive a complete assessment, which will help guide their treatment plan. Using the AEIOU-TIPS as a checklist of potential causes will help the EMT to determine what plan to follow or if ALS should be considered.

Stroke

According to the American Stroke Association, stroke is the fifth leading cause of death and disability in the United States, killing approximately 142,000 people a year. On average, someone suffers from a stroke every 40 seconds, so it is conceivable that an EMT will be called to a scene for "stroke-like symptoms."

Strokes are also called a cerebral vascular accident (CVA), which is when there is a sudden death of some brain cells due to lack of oxygen. This is when the blood flow to the brain is impaired by a blockage or rupture of an artery to the brain. The three main types of strokes are:

- **Ischemic** = caused by a blockage in a cerebral artery
- **Hemorrhagic** = when a blood vessel ruptures and bleeds freely
- **Transient Ischemic Attacks (TIA)** = "mini-stroke," which is a warning sign that a larger stroke will occur later in time

Whatever the cause of the stroke, signs and symptoms to pay attention to can be summarized in the acronym FAST (also known as the Cincinnati Prehospital Stroke Scale, or CPSS).

Pay attention to what is normal versus an abnormal response. If the patient gives an abnormal response, that is considered a positive sign for this scale, in which positive doesn't mean good, but rather that it is present in the patient at time of testing.

Table 6.5 *FAST Acronym to Describe Testing for Stroke-Like Symptoms*

Letter	What to Look For
F: Face	Ask the patient to smile. • Do both corners of the mouth turn upward, and equally? (*normal*) • Does it appear as if one side of the face is lower/unequal to the other side? • Is the patient's face numb? * Note that there is a condition called **Bell's palsy**, a temporary or permanent paralysis of a facial nerve, which may also cause facial droop. This is **not** a positive sign for stroke.
A: Arm drift	Ask the patient to raise both the arms up and in front, and hold them there for at least 5 seconds. • Is the patient able to hold both arms up without dropping down? (*normal*) • Is the patient able to lift only one arm and not the other?
S: Speech	Ask the patient to say a simple sentence such as "the sky is blue" and to then repeat it back to you. • Does the patient repeat back the words in the same order, without difficulty? (*normal*) • Does the patient repeat the words out of order? • Does the patient repeat back the same words or are they different? • Does the patient repeat back the sentence, but really struggle? • Does the patient slur the words? • Is the patient unable to speak?
T: Time	Ask the patient (or bystander) the following important questions: • When did the symptoms start? • When was the last time the patient was seen normal? • If this was a TIA where symptoms have resolved, how long did the symptoms last and with what frequency before EMS arrived?

Some medical practitioners add an additional two letters that describe additional symptoms to look out for, leading to the acronym BE FAST. However, the American Stroke Association still advocates for the scale as stated above.

- **B**: balance (have there been sudden balance issues?)
- **E**: eyes (has there been a sudden change or loss of vision in one or both eyes?)

There are additional stroke scales that are present in the medical world, and depending on where the EMT practices they may come upon them and be required to calculate a different stroke scale than listed above.

- **RACE**: Rapid Arterial Occlusion Evaluation
- **LAMS**: Los Angeles Motor Score
- **LAPSS**: Los Angeles Prehospital Stroke Screen
- **MEND**: Miami Emergency Neurological Deficit
- **NIHSS**: National Institutes of Health Stroke Scale

Whatever the scale used, as always, it is up to the EMT to know and understand the components that go into the stroke scale that their particular service or hospital prefers. Time is brain, so use it wisely.

Transient Ischemic Attacks (TIAs)

TIAs are a special type of stroke, often called a "mini-stroke." They are a temporary period of symptoms similar to those of an actual stroke. TIA symptoms usually last only a few minutes and don't cause permanent damage; many symptoms resolve completely within 24 hours. They are a warning sign—it may not happen that day or even that week, but it is a strong indicator of an impending cerebral vascular incident.

According to the Mayo Clinic, about one in three people who has a transient ischemic attack will eventually have a stroke, with about half occurring within a year after the TIA symptoms originally appeared.

The EMT may be called to a scene for stroke-like symptoms, yet upon arrival the patient presents with no deficits. However, the patient or a bystander may describe stroke symptoms that resolved prior to arrival, which leaves the EMT with little to test. However, this is not an excuse to sign a refusal and leave without doing a proper assessment and thorough questioning. In fact, it would be a great idea to convince the patient to transport to the hospital for further assessment, which patients may be reluctant to do if they believe they are now asymptomatic.

Shock and Sepsis

The Many Forms of Shock

Shock is best defined as inadequate perfusion and blood flow to the body's peripheral tissues, which leads to cellular and tissue hypoxia if not corrected. Perfusion, or the act of delivering oxygenated red blood cells to tissues and organs, requires an intact cardiovascular and respiratory system. If there is a breakdown within either system, shock will occur.

With this in mind, there are mainly four broad categories of shock listed in the table that follows. These are either caused by a pump, vessel, or fluid problem.

Table 6.6 *Types of Shock*

Type of Shock	Description and Examples
Distributive Shock	Fluid problem as a result of vasodilation and increased or decreased movement of fluids (typically blood) • Anaphylaxis: allergens trigger widespread vasodilation and movement of fluid out of the blood into the tissues • Neurogenic: sudden loss of the sympathetic nervous system signals to the smooth muscle in vessel walls, causing a drop in vascular resistance and hypotension • Sepsis: widespread infection travels via the blood throughout the body
Hypovolemic Shock	Fluid problem marked by loss of adequate volumes to keep the heart beating properly • Blood from trauma (internal or external) • Blood from nontraumatic injuries (ulcers, GI bleed) • Excessive vomiting • Burns and fluid shifts • Diarrhea • Excessive perspiration (sweating)
Cardiogenic Shock	Pump problem caused by the malfunction or cessation of the heart to beat • Myocardial infarction • Trauma such as myocardial contusion • Metabolic disorders that cause arrythmias • Pulmonary embolism located in the pulmonary vessels leading from the heart
Obstructive Shock	Vessel and pump problem caused when the normal flow of blood is obstructed • Cardiac tamponade (prevents blood from entering the heart) • Pneumothorax (increased pressure within the thoracic cavity blocks the flow) • Pulmonary embolism (a blockage in the pulmonary vessels which impedes blood flow back into the heart) • Plaque buildup or a piece that traveled from elsewhere in the body into a cardiac vessel, blocking normal blood flow

There are also multiple stages of shock a patient can experience.

Table 6.7 *Stages of Shock*

Stage of Shock	Signs and Symptoms
Stage 1 (compensated)	Occurs when the body first senses something is wrong and attempts to self-correct by doing the following: • Heart starts to beat faster • Blood vessels vasoconstrict • Respiratory rate increases to bring in more oxygen The patient may or may not be symptomatic, but with quick recognition and aggressive treatment reversal of this stage is very possible.
Stage 2 (decompensated)	Occurs when the natural compensation mechanisms begin to fail. Reversing this stage is not impossible but treatment must be aggressive. • Falling blood pressure (systolic of 90 mm Hg or lower with adults) • Weak, thready, or absent peripheral pulses • Decreasing mental status • Tachycardia and tachypnea • Skin color changes: pallor, ashy, cyanotic
Stage 3 (irreversible shock)	Occurs when poor perfusion has existed long enough to cause permanent damage to the body's organs and tissues. Cellular death is occurring systemically, and death is the ultimate conclusion.

Sepsis (The Silent Shock)

Sepsis is a cascade of inappropriate immune responses to the presence of an infection in the blood. It can lead to tissue damage, organ failure, amputations, and death.

Sepsis is the third leading cause of death in the United States. There are over 1.5 million cases per year, with nearly 270,000 deaths. Additionally, 1 in 3 hospital deaths is caused by sepsis.

This means that the EMT must be aware of the signs and symptoms, as they may very well come into contact with patients experiencing this progressive condition. It is especially prevalent in nursing homes or those who are immunocompromised, but in reality it transcends all demographics.

For the following table, EMS systems will primarily take BLS vital signs (and not blood work).

Table 6.8 *Diagnosis of Sepsis*

Tiered Level	Criteria
SIRS—Systemic Inflammation Response Syndrome	Need 2 or more to be considered positive: • HR above 90 per minute • Temperature higher than 100.4°F (38.6°C) or below 96.8°F (36°C) • RR above 20 per minute
SIRS + Source of infection = SEPSIS	Any sign of infection (external or internal) • Does the patient have any wounds? • Does the patient have pneumonia or another previously diagnosed bacterial infection? • Is the patient currently taking antibiotics, and if so, for what purpose?
Severe Sepsis	Sepsis + 1 or more of the following: • Systolic blood pressure less than 90 mm Hg or a drop greater than 40 mm Hg • Organ dysfunction • Hypoperfusion (shock) symptoms
Septic Shock	Severe sepsis + persistent hypotension despite adequate fluid resuscitation (*done by ALS or hospital personnel)

Many EMS systems have now implemented the ability to call a "sepsis alert" in the prehospital radio report. It is similar to calling in your regular radio report but adding that you believe your patient meets sepsis criteria. It has been statistically proven that sepsis alerts result in patients receiving faster blood testing and specific treatments aimed at stopping or slowing the cascade down.

EMS plays a vital role in delivering crucial information that ultimately will streamline the process of definitive patient care, which leads to a better outcome overall.

Diabetes, Seizures, and Allergies

Diabetes

Diabetes mellitus (DM) is a disease of the endocrine system that inhibits the body's ability to metabolize sugar. The organ that is responsible for insulin production is the pancreas, specifically in the islets of Langerhans cells. If these cells are impaired or damaged, insulin production will be affected.

Patients may or may not be on chronic medications that are either delivered by injection or in tablet or capsule format. Many patients who check their own blood glucose levels (BGL) using a glucometer on a daily basis are knowledgeable about their condition and can answer questions for the EMT.

The normal range of blood sugar is 80–120 mg/dL, although the range in patients with chronic diabetes may be much wider before physical symptoms occur.

The following table describes the various types of diabetes.

Table 6.9 *Types of Diabetes*

Type of Diabetes	Key Facts
Type I (juvenile diabetes or insulin dependent diabetes mellitus [IDDM])	• Less common (5–10% of diabetic patients) • Typically diagnosed in adolescence but can appear at any age • Results from the pancreas producing little to no insulin • Requires lifelong medication management by daily injections of insulin or by utilizing an insulin pump
Type II (adult-onset or insulin-resistant diabetes)	• More common • Chronic condition that affects the way the body processes blood sugar • Body produces insufficient amounts of insulin or it resists insulin • May be "cured" or effectively managed by making lifestyle changes such as healthier diet and exercise • Patients may take pills or capsules, rather than injectable insulin
Gestational Diabetes	• Diagnosed during pregnancy and may resolve after delivery • Some women may take insulin, but not all • Often causes baby to be extra large • Patients are more prone to hypertension or hypoglycemic events • Patients are at higher risk of developing type II diabetes later in life
Prediabetes	• Blood sugar level is higher than it should be but not high enough for the doctor to diagnose type II diabetes • All ages and genders can be affected • Lifestyle changes can reverse or halt progression • Patients are typically asymptomatic • One possible sign is darkened skin on certain parts of the body such neck, armpits, elbows, knees, and knuckles

Hypoglycemia

Hypoglycemia presents when blood sugar levels drop below 70–80 mg/dL. This is most often caused by taking the prescribed dosage of insulin and not following up with the regular ingestion of food as prescribed, causing the blood sugar to drop. On the other hand, the patient may have missed an insulin dosage or have not eaten a meal recently. Some additional causes could be vomiting, unusual exercise, and ingestion of alcohol. Any of these can cause the patient to either behave strangely or suddenly become unconscious.

Treatment at the BLS level includes oral glucose, oxygen, shock management, and rapid transport if symptoms do not improve or they are unresponsive/unconscious. Follow your local protocols as indicated.

Signs and symptoms include:

- Shakiness/dizziness
- Irritability, anxiety, nervousness, combativeness
- Hunger
- Headache
- Slurred words/altered mental status/confusion
- Muscle weakness
- Blurred vision
- Staggered gait
- Clammy or diaphoretic skin
- Convulsions or seizures

Hyperglycemia

Defined as high blood sugar, hyperglycemia doesn't cause symptoms until glucose values are significantly elevated—usually above 180–200 mg/dL. Some glucometers will just state "high," which could indicate levels of 400–600 mg/dL.

Treatment at the BLS levels includes shock management, oxygen if indicated, and rapid transport if symptoms do not improve or become worse. ALS intervention may also be indicated for airway and cardiac management. Follow your local protocols as indicated.

Signs and symptoms include:

- Frequent thirst (polydipsia)
- Frequent urination (polyuria)
- Increased hunger (polyphagia)
- A fruity odor on the breath (ketone production)
- Shortness of breath or tachypnea

The longer blood sugar levels stay high, the more serious the symptoms become and can lead to conditions such as diabetic ketoacidosis or DKA.

Patients may wear a Medic Alert™ bracelet (or other medical jewelry), which identifies them as having this condition. When doing an assessment of the patient, look for any jewelry of this type to save time and help you develop a more rapid treatment plan.

It may also help you advocate on the patient's behalf, especially in the presence of law enforcement or other bystanders who may not understand the symptoms of hypoglycemia.

Treatment is as follows:

- Most state protocols will allow the EMT to administer oral **glucose** to patients who present with these symptoms and are conscious. If the condition is the result of hypoglycemia, the patient will usually respond very quickly to the oral sugar.
- Some state protocols will allow the EMT to administer **glucagon** via intramuscular injection. Glucagon is a protein that causes sugar stored in the liver to be released into the bloodstream (and consequently is ineffective in patients with chronic liver disease, such as cirrhosis or hepatitis).

Not all states allow glucagon administration at the BLS level, and it is not included in the EMT National Curriculum. However, as each state is independent in making its own protocols, this may be allowed as indicated.

Glucometer Usage

Many states now allow basic EMS units to carry portable glucometers that enable the EMT to accurately gauge the blood glucose level (BGL). This may be especially important to the treating physician, as it will give a baseline blood sugar reading prior to any intervention by EMS.

Patients may also have their own glucometers, and you can use their reading to compare to your own results. Be aware that different manufacturers have different reading thresholds so there may be slight variances in numerical results.

To check the BGL level, follow these steps:

1. Gather your materials: glucometer, collecting strips, lancet, alcohol prep pad, gauze pad, and adhesive bandage.
2. Insert the collection strip into the glucometer and make sure that the machine is ready to collect the blood, typically shown with a blood drop icon.
3. Select the finger you will use to collect blood; clean the fingertip with the alcohol prep pad for at least 15 seconds.

4. Remove the safety mechanism of the lancet so that the needle is ready to deploy.

5. Holding the finger still, press the lancet (needle side down) onto the fleshy part of the underside or lateral side of the finger, deploying the needle.

6. Wipe away the first drop of blood with the gauze pad.

7. Gently squeeze the finger to produce fresh blood and place the collecting strip directly into the blood drop; make sure the blood is drawn up completely into the strip and the glucometer indicates it is reading the results.

8. Place a band-aid onto the finger and read the glucometer results; record them in your documentation.

9. Throw away any trash produced and place the used lancet into the sharps container.

Seizures

Seizures, or involuntary muscular activity, may be caused by many things, such as high fever, hypoglycemia, head injury, or brain disease (e.g., epilepsy). They are seen in all ages and genders. The EMT may be called while a seizure is occurring or just after it has ended.

Seizure activity falls into two main categories—generalized onset and focal onset. Generalized onset affects both sides of the brain or groups of cells on both sides of the brain at the same time. Focal onset can start in one area or group of cells in one side of the brain.

Keep in mind that as neuroscience progresses, there may be more categories or types of seizures being named or refined into categories. The following table attempts to list the more common type of seizure activity the EMT may be called to assist with.

Table 6.10 *Types of Seizure*

Seizure Category	Types of Seizure
Generalized Onset Seizure	• Absence (formally known as *petit-mal*) • Tonic-clonic (formally known as *grand-mal*) • Atonic (no shaking, only muscle weakness) • Febrile (caused by high fever, typically in children) • Status epilepticus
Focal Onset Seizure	• Simple focal (also known as simple partial) • Complex focal (also known as a complex partial) • Myoclonic (sudden movements lasting less than a few seconds at a time)

Absence seizure causes rapid blinking or a few seconds of staring into space. Typically, the person may not even realize that seizure activity took place and it is noticed instead by a bystander. A person may have multiple episodes in a day.

Tonic-clonic seizure (type most familiar to people) has two phases: in the tonic portion the body becomes rigid, and in the clonic portion there is uncontrollable jerking motion. Episodes may last a few seconds or several minutes. A person may finish one seizure and have another one shortly afterward.

Prolonged seizure (known as status epilepticus) is a true medical emergency, since patients will begin to develop a lack of oxygen to the brain that could result in brain damage or brain death. This condition is defined as a continuous seizure lasting more than 30 minutes, or two or more seizures without full recovery of consciousness between any of them. This is why it is vitally important to ask the patient or bystanders how long the seizure activity lasted and record their answer.

Most seizures are of short duration, and the active portion of the seizure has usually subsided when EMS arrives on the scene. Seizures are followed by a period of unconsciousness or semi-consciousness referred to as the *postictal phase*. In this phase, the patient may be confused, possibly combative, or take longer to answer questions than what is typically considered baseline for them. Be patient, as this phase can last from 5–30 minutes or longer depending on the person.

Treatment of the seizure patient is as follows:

Table 6.11 *BLS Seizure Treatment*

Phase	BLS Treatment
Actively Seizing	• Request ALS, as they have medications to help control seizures • Move the patient to a safe area or clear away any objects nearby, especially near the head (that the patient could strike) • Have suction ready, as the airway may become compromised • Give the patient high flow oxygen via NRB, from 12–15 lpm, to help with increased consumption by the brain • Do not attempt to stick anything in or remove (prior) objects from the patient's mouth • If this is not a chronic problem for the patient, you may have to provide emotional support for family members or bystanders, who may never have witnessed a seizure and are confused; it can be frightening • Be prepared for recurrence • Make the decision to stay on scene vs. transport, especially if ALS is farther away than the hospital
Postictal	• Be prepared to ventilate or clear the airway if necessary • If the patient remains confused for longer than 20 minutes after a seizure, consider another cause of AMS and call ALS if indicated • Ask how long each seizure lasted, how many they had, and what they were doing before the seizure happened • Administer oxygen via NRB at 12–15 lpm if you haven't already done so

Transport of the seizure patient follows the usual pattern of assuring a patent airway and placing the patient on his side (recumbent) in the event of vomiting. If the EMT cannot rule out the possibility of trauma, then the patient is secured with a cervical collar, head blocks, and a spine board to guard against spinal cord injury. The patient is then transported supine and the entire board is rolled in the event of vomiting.

Remember that seizures may be caused by head trauma, and a GCS score would be appropriate in this scenario.

Allergic Reaction

An allergic reaction is an exaggerated immune-system response by the body to a substance. The most common substances that cause allergies are insect bites/stings, nuts, shellfish, medications, and certain plants. However, any substance can be an allergen, depending on the body's response to it.

A possible allergic reaction (anaphylaxis) should be suspected if the patient reports tingling and heat in the face, mouth, or extremities, severe itching, visible hives, flushed skin, and swelling to the extremities. The main concern is to ensure that the airway does not swell shut and prevent the patient from breathing; therefore, dispatches to possible allergic reactions are always treated as priority calls.

Other symptoms of anaphylaxis may include:

- Chest tightness and pressure
- Prolonged uncontrolled coughing
- Tachypnea
- Dyspnea
- Hoarseness, stridor, audible wheezing
- Rapid pulse rate
- Low blood pressure (as the body attempts to regulate its response to the allergen)

If the reactions include altered mental status, then hypoxia and hypoperfusion may be severe, and immediate treatment is indicated.

After you perform an initial assessment and treat any necessary conditions, proceed to the focused assessment. There you must be alert to any history of past allergic reactions, the events that immediately preceded the symptoms that prompted the call to the EMS system, and whether those events were related to past allergic reactions.

Food allergies may be particularly insidious in this regard. For example, a person with a severe allergy to nuts will avoid nuts, but nut by-products may be used in the processing of other foods and may cause a surprise reaction.

Treatment is, first, a complete focused assessment, baseline vital signs, and the administration of oxygen. If the patient is having difficulty breathing, epinephrine is indicated. If the patient is not symptomatic and breathing adequately, you may see if there is a visible injection site. If you do, scraping away the stinger is indicated and can be done using a credit card or similar item. Be careful not to use tweezers when trying to remove a stinger as it could inadvertently squeeze a venom sac that may still be attached to the end of it.

If epinephrine is indicated, it will reverse the effects of severe anaphylaxis long enough to transport the patient to a medical facility. It constricts the blood vessels and increases the heart rate to help raise the blood pressure and combat hypoperfusion syndrome.

- See if the patient is carrying an epinephrine syringe. If yes, the patient should have been instructed in its usage and administration route, perhaps even administering it prior to the EMT's arrival.
  - Some jurisdictions allow the EMT to administer an epinephrine syringe after consulting medical control if patients have not already done so or have had no relief with the first injection.
  - Check the 5 Rights before administering.
- After administration, reassess the patient and note any changes in her condition.
  - If the patient had trouble breathing and airway swelling earlier, and both have responded to the epinephrine, then that usually confirms the assessment of anaphylaxis.
- Advise the receiving facility of the outcome of your intervention.

Anaphylaxis often begins as dyspnea, so airway management is the most important condition to be managed.

Poisoning and Overdose

A poison is defined as any substance that produces harmful physiological or psychological effects to the body. According to the National Safety Council, poisoning is responsible for approximately 10% of all emergency department admissions in the United States. Overdose is when serious physiological and psychological effects occur from the overuse or misuse of any substance by exceeding safe dosages. The substance may be a legal substance, such as alcohol, or an illegal substance, such as cocaine or heroin.

The stereotypical poisoning case is that of the child who gets into the cleaning supplies beneath the sink, a relatively infrequent EMS dispatch. In reality, most EMTs deal with a large number of calls involving either alcohol overdose or the use of illegal drugs.

Poisons may enter the body in a variety of ways.

- **Ingestion** is when the substance is taken by mouth, such as drinking a toxic substance or taking pills.
- **Inhalation** is when the substance is inhaled into the lungs, such as breathing in poisons like carbon monoxide from car exhaust in a closed space or snorting cocaine.
- **Injection** involves placing the substance directly into the bloodstream using a hypodermic syringe, as with injecting heroin.
- **Absorption** occurs when toxins enter the body by contact with the skin, such as with poison ivy or pesticide poisoning.

Signs and symptoms of poisoning will vary depending on the poison and how the body reacts to it. The EMT must be prepared to intervene if there is a sudden change in the patient's condition and to perform basic life support functions as needed. If good scene and patient assessments are done, the EMT may know what the specific poison is and be in a better position to begin treatment while en route to the emergency department. A resource that is available to both the public and medical professionals, including EMS, is poison control. There are national numbers as well as state-run hotlines. They are available 24 hours a day, 7 days a week, and can help guide treatment for both ALS and BLS providers alike.

Scene Assessment

The EMT should be proactive in trying to determine why the patient is presenting with specific symptoms, as that knowledge may well be the difference between a successful outcome and sudden patient death.

- If you arrive at the scene of a woman down, unconscious in her bed, with bradypnea, bradycardia, pale and diaphoretic and unresponsive, she could be the victim of a number of medical problems.
- If you notice an empty pill bottle of Percocet™ next to the bed, you may suspect an opioid overdose and notify the receiving facility of this finding, which will expedite treatment in the ER.

Without that initial assessment, the receiving facility would have to perform a wide range of initial tests and potentially lose critical time.

If you are unsure of a medication name, use reference material or do a quick online search on your cell phone to identify the drug. Be sure to use a medically oriented, verified source, and not just any popular website.

Another part of a complete assessment is to bring to the receiving facility any identifying containers or labels. These may contain the chemical information necessary for treatment, as well as indicate the amount of the poison ingested by the patient.

Treatment

Treatment of suspected poisoning will follow the usual protocol of assessing and treating the basic life-support functions. If the poison is known, basic protocols may allow treatments in the prehospital setting with proper medical control.

- Activated charcoal (oral administration), depending on the poison and the amount of time since ingestion
  - Activated charcoal is ground charcoal in a suspension of water, forming aqueous slurry.
  - May cause vomiting but is otherwise benign.
- Naloxone (or Narcan), an opioid-reversal (antagonist) medication (used routinely in EMS)
  - Can be delivered intranasal (IN) or intramuscular (IM) by BLS
  - Dosage for IN: 2 mg/mL (1 mg per nostril)
  - Dosage for IM: 0.4 mg/0.4 mL in lateral thigh
  - Protocol will dictate how many, if any, repeat dosages can be given by the EMT

If the patient is actively vomiting (or has previously done so), this is more problematic if the poison is caustic, corrosive, or a petroleum product. These poisons will cause more damage to the esophageal passage as they come back up, and thus are better treated by being neutralized in the stomach. Petroleum products may also cause problems in the lungs if their vapors are aspirated.

Syrup of ipecac, which is still sold in pharmacies today, is not used in EMS routinely and is not included in the National Curriculum for EMTs as a standard medication.

Emergency care for poisoning and overdose involves good basic life support: maintaining an airway, adequate oxygen perfusion, and circulatory support, if necessary. A complete initial assessment followed by a comprehensive focused assessment is crucial to good prehospital care. As always, scene safety is crucial.

- In the case of bee sting, if the bees are still swarming, then the scene is not safe and should not be entered unless the EMT is wearing suitable protective equipment. If the EMT is safe, then the patient must be removed as expeditiously as possible from the unsafe condition.

- In the case of carbon-monoxide poisoning, the EMT must be aware of the lethality of the odorless gas in a closed space. If the scene is safe, the EMT can transport the poisoned individual to a receiving facility with a hyperbaric chamber, a device helpful in carbon-monoxide poisoning.

Environmental Emergencies

In order to function properly, the human body consistently maintains an average internal temperature of ~98.6°F.

Note that the key word is *average* in the previous sentence. Some people may normally run a slightly lower or higher internal temperature as their baseline and be nonsymptomatic or in distress. However, for diagnostic purposes, most medical professionals use 98.6°F or 37°C as the starting point.

When writing or reading temperatures, the letter F is shorthand for Fahrenheit while C is shorthand for Celsius. The United States is one of the few countries in the world that uses Fahrenheit as its standard of measurement, so if you come across something written in Celsius you may have to convert it in the field.

Core temperature is considered the most accurate, and that is achieved with a rectal (internal) thermometer. However, since that isn't practical, most EMS systems use an oral, tympanic (ear), or axillary (armpit) type.

In a hot or cold emergency, energy may be transferred in a variety of ways.

Table 6.12 *Pathways of Heat Energy Transfer*

Type of Energy Transfer	Key Facts
Radiation	• Heat is given off into an area or object that has a lower temperature than the radiating object • Example: a person standing outdoors in subfreezing temperatures radiates heat to the surrounding cold atmosphere, primarily through the extremities
Convection	• Heat or energy is transferred through a fluid (gas or liquid) from high temperature to low temperature by molecular movement • Example: when blood circulates, heat is generated by the cells in the body and then transferred to air or water that is flowing over the skin (explains why we will feel chilly if a cooler wind blows over our arms when we are sweating)
Conduction	• Heat is passed through a colder object by direct contact • Example: water will conduct heat 240 times faster than air, which is why a subject immersed in cold water is subject to rapid hypothermia
Evaporation	• Liquid is heated to a gaseous state, causing a loss of temperature • Example: the process of perspiring (sweating) is one of the regulatory mechanisms the body uses to maintain normal temperature

Hypothermia

Hypothermia (heat loss) is a loss of body temperature. It is a commonly seen situation in emergency medicine. The EMT might respond to a patient in a cold environment without suitable clothing or someone who has been rapidly immersed into cold water. Especially susceptible to this condition are the extremely young and the extremely old.

There are three levels of hypothermia a patient can experience:

- **Mild**: core temperature 90–95°F (32–35°C)
- **Moderate**: core temperature 82–90°F (28–32°C)
- **Severe**: core temperature below 82°F (28°C)

Studies have shown that exposed flesh will freeze in less than 1 minute at −70°F. While this temperature is not common in the continental United States, that has the same effect as −20°F + a wind of 25–30 mph, a common winter condition in the northern United States.

Gradual hypothermia progresses through five stages:

- **Stage 1**: The body shivers as it attempts to raise its core temperature by the activity
- **Stage 2**: Mental apathy and loss of motor functions begin to occur
- **Stage 3**: Decreased level of responsiveness; freezing of the extremities
- **Stage 4**: Vital signs begin to decrease and slow
- **Stage 5**: Death

Assessment of hypothermia by the EMT includes the following:

- Feel the patient's torso or abdomen, which will be the best indicator for a low core body temperature.
- If it feels cold to the touch, check verbal and motor responses and note whether they are normal or impaired (and if so, to what degree).
- If shivering is present, then the patient may be in stage 1. If shivering is absent, the patient may already be in stage 2 or 3.
- As hypothermia progresses, skin color will initially be red, then pale, and finally cyanotic or black. It will also become stiff and hard in the advanced stages.

Treatment of hypothermia starts with removal from the cold environment and removal of any wet clothing.

- Warm patient gradually with blankets and warm water bottles or hot packs to the groin, axillary, and cervical regions.
- Raise the ambient temperature of the truck as the patient is transported.
- Give supplemental oxygen at the highest level that the patient can tolerate.

Localized cold injuries, or frostbite, will begin in the extremities and in any areas with poor circulation. The skin will initially turn white and progress to a waxy look as the injury progresses. It will feel frozen and rigid upon palpation, and swelling and blisters may be present.

- Gradually rewarm the extremity (use warm water bath if there is a long or delayed transport).
- The patient will complain of severe pain as the injured extremity begins to thaw.
- To minimize long-term damage of the extremity, splinting may be needed.

Hyperthermia

Hyperthermia is abnormally high body temperature. Heat gained exceeds heat lost, which can lead to a potentially fatal increase in the core body temperature.

Table 6.13 *Heat Emergencies*

Type of Hyperthermia	Key Facts and Treatment
Heat Cramps	• Muscle cramps caused by excessive body heat; not always due to strenuous activity • Usually the first indicator of hyperthermia • Treat by cooling the patient gradually
Heat Exhaustion	• General weakness accompanied by warm skin and profuse sweating • To transport, remove to a cooler environment and place in a semi-Fowler position • Treat by cooling the patient gradually and increasing the air-conditioning
Heat Stroke	• Severe hyperthermia caused by a failure of the body's cooling mechanism • **Onset of altered mental status** (main difference between heat exhaustion and heatstroke) • Skin might be hot + dry or hot + sweaty • Treated by cooling the patient aggressively, with cold, wet towels or ice packs to the groin, axillary, and cervical regions (done en route to the emergency department, i.e., do not delay transport)

Water Emergencies

Water emergencies present their own unique set of challenges to the EMT. Scene safety is always paramount, with the following guidelines:

- No rescue should ever be attempted that is beyond your skill level.
- Initial attempts should be made to throw an object or flotation device to the victim.
- On open waters, attempt to use a boat if one is available.
- As a last resort, swimming out to a victim who is drowning should be undertaken only by a suitably trained rescuer.

As with any situation where the mechanism of injury is unknown, assume that the victim has suffered a traumatic injury and take the suitable spinal precautions. If the victim is breathing and has a pulse, consider placement on a spine board while still in the water.

- A victim who has been immersed in cold water and who presents with no breathing or pulse should be given CPR immediately, as the mammalian diving reflex may have taken effect.
- A victim who has been in the water for less than 1 hour should receive resuscitation efforts. (In colder weather, patients have been resuscitated up to 2 hours after being submerged.)

If there is a problem ventilating a patient due to abdominal distention, the patient should be placed left lateral recumbent and gentle pressure should be applied to the abdomen to relieve the distention. Suction should be ready to assist in clearing the airway if fluid is vomited by this maneuver.

All mammals, including humans, have the **mammalian diving reflex**. The body has an innate physiological response to submersion in cold water. It selectively shuts down parts of the body, conserving oxygen while maintaining homeostasis within the body.

Drowning Emergencies

According to the World Health Organization (WHO), drowning is the third leading cause of unintentional injury-related death worldwide, accounting for 7% of all injury-related deaths. Children, people who have increased contact with water, and males statistically are the most at risk for drowning incidents.

Studies suggest that the higher drowning rates among males are due to increased exposure to water and riskier behavior such as swimming alone, drinking alcohol before or during water activities, and boating accidents.

Children typically have drowning emergencies due to either lack of supervision or accidental falls into a body of water. In fact, statistics show that drowning is the leading cause of death in children ages 1–4, with children 5–9 not far behind.

Anywhere there is a body of water that can allow for submersion of a head or body is at risk for having a drowning incident. This can include buckets, bathtubs, pools, lakes, or even showers!

Treatment is the same regardless of what caused the drowning—if artificial respirations are required, they must be performed with adequate tidal volume and rate. If CPR is indicated, make sure the patient is out of the body of water and onto a hard surface for compressions. Make sure the chest is wiped clean of water before using an AED. Have suction ready to go for secretions or any water that may come up. If traumatic injuries are present, manage them appropriately. Finally, be prepared for hypothermia and shock management.

Diving Emergencies

While not always a common call, diving emergencies must be thoroughly explored by asking good assessment questions such as:

- "How long did it take the diver to ascend to the surface, and did he stop along the way?"
- "How deep and long was the dive?"
- "How long was it before the diver showed signs or symptoms?"
- "What type of breathing gas was the diver using?"

Table 6.14 *Diving Emergencies and Systems Affected*

Affected System	Issues That Can Arise
Temperature	• Needs to be regulated; certain types of clothing or protective gear can help or hinder this • In cold water, the body could automatically gasp for breath, which could escalate into hyperventilation and drowning • Heat loss and gain, plus dehydration can occur
Cardiac	• Immersion into water (especially cold) can cause arrhythmias leading to syncope or death • Nervousness or fright may cause tachypnea or tachycardia, especially if the diver is inexperienced

Respiratory	• In cold water temperatures, the body could automatically gasp for breath, which could escalate into hyperventilation and drowning
	• Expanding air due to pressure changes may rupture the lung and cause a pneumothorax
	   – Subcutaneous emphysema can result from air that escapes
	   – Air emboli may travel to or from the brain, causing syncope or stroke-like symptoms
	• Pressure changes can cause injury to ears and sinuses

Musculoskeletal	• Nitrogen can be forced into or released from tissues, depending on descent or ascent ("the bends"); the result is pain and death if not corrected • Traumatic injuries can occur if struck by objects or animals underwater

Treatment includes thorough questioning, removing the patient from the environment using safety or possible spinal precautions, disconnecting equipment that will be in the provider's way, providing oxygen as necessary and indicated, and transport to the hospital.

Some divers may require a hyperbaric chamber, which can reduce the pressure inside the body in a safe, controlled manner, but these chambers are not available at all hospitals. Refer to your local protocols for guidance and potential identification of such facilities.

Bites and Stings

Bites and stings are treated as both wounds and possible injection poisonings. In addition, there is always the possibility of an allergic reaction.

Never attempt to "suck" out any venom with your mouth or the patient's. A tourniquet or pressure bandage above or below can help stop spread of the venom. The EMT may also wish to draw a circle around the bite using a pen or marker, to help determine if swelling or skin redness is growing by comparing the circle drawn to where the outside edges of the swelling or redness is located en route. Transport to the most appropriate hospital or if available in your service area, to a hospital that has an envenomation specialist on staff.

If there is bleeding associated with the wound, control the bleeding as necessary using sterile gauze and bandages. Remember to always check and reassess pulse, motor function, and sensory abilities when bandaging any wounds.

If appropriate and indicated by local protocol, consider the usage of epinephrine and oxygen if respiratory symptoms are present.

Unless specifically directed by local protocol, do not attempt to collect or capture the animal that caused the bite or sting. You could injure yourself, plus you would have to find a place to dispose of the animal (especially if it is still alive). Contact animal control or similar services to perform this task if necessary.

Keep good documentation, however, of the type of animal that caused the injury; this could be helpful information in treatment decisions at the hospital, as well as in your own run report.

Height and Climbing Emergencies

Activities such as climbing at high elevations may involve emergencies requiring EMS assistance.

- Thermal emergency (hyperthermia/hypothermia), especially if wearing inappropriate clothing for the activity pursuing
- Musculoskeletal trauma, such as a twisted ankle, broken hand, shoulder dislocation, head injury, or spinal damage, if falling from a height
- Dehydration, due to thermal emergency or overexertion
- Exhaustion and/or confusion, which can be exacerbated if the patient has gotten lost and care has been delayed

Height matters with respect to documentation and also as a clue to the type of injury the person has suffered. Consider the following guidelines:

- Report ground level falls as zero (0) feet.
- If the patient has fallen from a natural object or ladder, use the distance from lowest part of the body to the ground/surface. For instance, if the patient fell from the 5-inch step of a ladder, the fall was 5 inches. If the patient fell from a 12-foot tree onto the grass, the fall was 12 feet.
- Look for injury patterns that are not obvious visual injuries. With falls from heights, even if landing on the feet, energy can transfer from the feet, up the spine, and into other parts of the body, causing damage. Internal bones can become fractured, as well. Use spinal precautions as directed by local protocols.

Behavioral Emergencies

When an emergency doesn't fall into the category of a police situation or fire emergency, the default agency called is EMS. That includes what are called "behavioral emergencies," i.e., situations involving patients with psychiatric or emotional emergencies.

In the early days of EMS, there was very little training for patients with psychiatric or emotional problems, even though EMS was the lead agency called. As a result, many EMS treatment protocols were developed over time, "after the fact."

The National Standard Curriculum mandates that the EMT be able to define *behavior* and *behavioral emergency*.

- **Behavior** is defined as the "manner in which a person acts or performs; any or all activities of a person, including physical and mental activity."
- **Behavioral emergency** is defined as "a situation in which the patient exhibits abnormal behavior within a given situation that is unacceptable or intolerable to the patient, family, or community." Causes include:
  - Extremes of emotion, leading to violence or other inappropriate behavior
  - A psychological or physical condition such as lack of oxygen or low blood sugar in diabetes

Some behaviors are obviously unacceptable or intolerable. Threatening to commit suicide or threatening to violently assault another person are clear examples. These may be conscious, rational decisions, or they may be brought on by certain medical conditions in otherwise healthy individuals:

- Low blood sugar
- Anoxia
- Inadequate blood perfusion to the brain
- Head trauma
- Mind-altering substance
- Psychosis
- Excessive heat/cold

The key words in the definition of behavioral emergency are "unacceptable" or "intolerable." This is oftentimes a subjective determination. A person walking down the street naked and singing may be acceptable in a nudist camp, but in any metropolitan area would likely be arrested or require EMS intervention.

Be aware of the standards of behavior in the community in which you practice.

The good news is that most behavioral emergency calls are usually nonviolent. A patient may have a panic attack with a sudden irrational fear or may be crying and unable to stop. But some patients with mental illness may become violent, so you must be prepared to react quickly to ensure a safe environment for all, leading to the proper treatment of the patient.

Common Psychological Crises

There are common psychological crises that EMS may encounter on the job. Any of these crises may pose a danger to the patient (increased risk of bodily harm due to risky or suicidal behavior) or to bystanders and responding EMTs.

Table 6.15 *Common Behavioral Emergencies*

Psychological Issue	Definition and Manifestations
Anxiety or Panic Disorder	• **Agitation or unreasonable fear of current or future events** • Tachypnea, tachycardia, numbness/tingling of the extremities • Mistrust of the provider • Low oxygen saturation levels if hyperventilating
Phobia(s)	• **Irrational fear of (specific) things, places, or situations** • Hallucinations (auditory or visual) • Tachypnea, tachycardia • Mistrust of the provider or bystanders
Depression	• **Deep feelings of sadness, worthlessness, and discouragement with no sign of any relief** • Flat affect (monotone voice or animation of body) • Suicidal thoughts • Risky behavior such as use of illegal drugs, excessive alcohol consumption, or self-harm, i.e., cutting or burning their skin • Lack of desire to eat, drink, or do daily activities of living such as showering or cleaning • Noncompliance with medication
Bipolar Disorder	• **Mood of extreme euphoria alternating with extreme depression** (stages may last a few minutes to months at a time) • Risky behaviors seen with depression (above) • Suicidal or homicidal thoughts • Elevated vital signs if in a manic episode • Noncompliance with medication used as mood stabilizers
Paranoia	• **Chronic and deep fear and mistrust of everyone and everything** • Mistrust of the provider • Elevated vital signs if anxious or agitated • Confusion or disjointed speech • Auditory or visual hallucinations

(Continued)

Table 6.15 *Common Behavioral Emergencies (Continued)*

Psychological Issue	Definition and Manifestations
Schizophrenia	• **Chronic and severe mental disorder that affects how a person thinks, feels, and behaves** • Delusions/hallucinations, disorganized speech or behavior, blunted or flat affect, thought disorders (unusual or dysfunctional ways of thinking), or catatonia • Poor "executive functioning" skills, i.e., the ability to understand information and use it to make decisions • Noncompliance with prescribed medication
Suicidal and Homicidal Thoughts	• **Thoughts to harm oneself or others, with or without a clear plan to do so; may or may not be an underlying mental illness** • Flat affect or speech patterns • Refusal to be transported (especially if someone else called 911) • A collection of items that could be used to harm: guns, excess of pills (prescription or not), ropes, knives • Depression or agitated mood
Excited Delirium	• **Typically caused by illicit stimulant drug usage or underlying mental illness; often first experienced in prehospital setting** • Sudden onset • Bizarre and/or aggressive behavior; shouting or verbal agitation • Paranoia or panic • Violence toward others • Unexpected and strong physical strength • Hyperthermia, even up to 102°F or higher

As part of securing the scene and patient assessment, be alert for patients who pace nervously, shout, threaten others, curse, throw objects, or stand grimacing with clenched fists. A patient exhibiting any of these signs should be presumed capable of a sudden violent attack. If a behavioral problem is ever suspected on one of your calls, police support should be available.

Suicidal Behavior

This category of behavioral emergencies requires special mention. The EMT may be called out for "suicidal ideation" or an unknown behavioral emergency that turns out to be a suicide attempt. Some patients are very honest and seek assistance, in which case your empathy and care can be of enormous help. Other patients, such as a severely depressed person, might decline medical intervention (which is their right unless they are impaired).

That said, a patient who is at an increased risk for suicide is presumed to "not have the capacity to refuse medical treatment." In other words:

- If the patient states somethings like, "I want to kill myself," you must insist on his transport (i.e., you must not allow him to refuse transport) to a medical facility.

- If a patient makes a vague reference to not wanting to be here anymore or something like, "Nobody would miss me anyway," you must decide whether the patient is actually at risk for a suicide attempt.

  - Ask clarifying questions to determine the true reason that 911 was called, either by the patient or a bystander.

  - If the patient has made suicidal comments, it is often helpful to repeat back the statement and ask if that is true or not. Do so with the idea of verifying information, not with judgment or hostility in your voice and body language.

- Indicators of an increased risk of suicide, and thus in determining if a patient cannot refuse transport, include the following:

  - Age >40 and single/widowed/divorced

  - History of alcohol abuse or illegal drug use

  - History of depression, especially if not medicated or receiving professional treatment

  - Individuals who have a defined lethal plan of action that they will verbalize

  - Unusual gathering of articles that can cause death, i.e., guns, pills, ropes

  - Previous history of suicide attempts/behaviors

  - Recently diagnosed serious illness

  - Recent loss of a loved one or relationship troubles

  - Recent arrest or imprisonment

  - Loss of job or financial security

As you assess a patient with any of these risk factors, be sure to present a calm yet authoritative demeanor.

- Maintain eye contact and speak in a measured, calm tone.

- If the patient questions you, answer honestly yet in a way that is noninflammatory. Rather than come across as "disagreeing" with the patient, try an approach that presents more positive alternatives, such as the concern of the patient's family.

- If the patient is delusional or hallucinating, assure him that the symptoms are not real.

Lastly, do not forget to properly document the patient's statements (even if they change), and report to hospital personnel.

Restraints

Behavioral calls are normally longer in duration than others, as the EMT often has to get the patient to cooperate in transportation to the medical facility. Yet in spite of all of the EMT's best efforts, it is sometimes necessary to forcibly restrain a patient.

Local protocols vary in the use of restraints. Some jurisdictions limit the application of restraints to police, some allow EMS to restrain patients with medical control approval, and others allow EMS to restrain if it can document a clear threat. Local protocols should always be followed, since the alternative may be a charge against the EMT for assault, battery, and/or false imprisonment.

Most services allow the use of soft restraints and have migrated away from the usage of leather or vinyl restraints. It is very rare for EMS services to allow the usage of handcuffs or zip ties, as that is often only handled by police officers.

Police may deliver patients to EMS with their wrists secured in handcuffs behind their backs and their ankles in leg irons (placing violent patients in a prone position is common for police). If a patient in this position is delivered into your care, you must immediately place him or her in a lateral recumbent position to preclude asphyxia.

If EMS is authorized to restrain a violent patient, then ideally, a minimum of five people are necessary for the safe application of soft restraints—one for each limb and one to apply the restraints. As it is not always possible for this number of people to be on scene initially, consider calling for additional assistance before attempting a restraint maneuver. Never attempt to restrain a patient without a clear plan in which every member of the team has verified they are clear on what their roles are. If this is not done, this is a sure recipe for disaster and can result in harm to the patient, as well as the EMS crew.

A patient should never be restrained in a prone position with ankles drawn up, the so-called "hog-tie." Many deaths due to asphyxia have been documented of patients in this type of restraint.

Securing a patient to a backboard requires the following steps:

1. With a person holding on each limb, the patient is forced into a supine position on a backboard.
2. Restraint cuffs are placed on each ankle and then secured to prevent kicking.
3. A strap is used to secure the patient's legs just above the knees.
4. Another strap is used across the chest just below the armpits.
5. A restraint cuff is applied to each wrist, and the arms are crossed over the chest and restrained to the backboard.

Alternatively, you could restrain the wrists with the nondominant hand (if known) tractioned along the side of the body and secure the dominant hand to the top of the backboard above the patient's head.

- The advantages to this method are that the patient's torso is clear. If chest compressions suddenly have to be performed, the EMT can observe the patient's diaphragm for signs of respiratory distress, and the patient's arm is available for an IV if one becomes necessary.

- The disadvantages are that the patient is less secure than with the arms crossed over the chest, since the arms would help to maintain the supine position.

Respiratory function and distal circulation should constantly be checked, as the patient could quickly become impaired because of the restraints.

Metal restraints (handcuffs and leg irons) have the potential to damage tendons and ligaments. However, since they are quick and easy to use, they can be safer than leather and vinyl restraints. The solution is to switch a patient in metal restraints to softer restraints once sufficient personnel can assist.

Another option is to secure the patient onto the stretcher mattress frame using the stretcher frame (not arm rail) as an anchoring point. Place restraint cuffs on each ankle and secure to prevent kicking. A restraint cuff is then applied to each wrist and secured to the stretcher frame as well. Any number of knots could be used to secure restraints that will minimize harm to the patient, while allowing you to effectively manage any safety concerns.

To reiterate, local medical protocols must always be followed. Behavioral emergencies, because of their medical and legal complexities, must be thoroughly documented, both as to observation of the patient and EMS interactions. Any medical-control permissions must be documented completely as to the individual giving permission for specific actions and the time of permission. Since complaints against EMTs are common in these situations, it is important that the names of witnesses, assisting EMT, and police officers are also well documented.

If a situation becomes unsafe, you must evacuate, call for additional help, and replan. Do not place yourself in serious danger trying to restrain someone.

Obstetric and Gynecological Emergencies

Childbirth is a natural process, and the EMT's role is one of support, as well as recognition of abnormal situations should they present. As with medical emergencies and trauma, the EMT must be aware of the special anatomy and physiology of the pregnant female and her unborn child.

Pregnancy and Childbirth

The fetus lives in the uterus, or womb, of the mother.

- Once a female's ovum (egg) is fertilized by a male sperm, it begins to grow and divide into multiple cells and implants itself in the wall of the uterus, where it will be nourished.
- The normal period for gestation is approximately 40 weeks from the time of ovum fertilization.
- The opening of the uterus into the birth canal, or vagina, is called the cervix. This opening is blocked by a mucus plug during pregnancy, which is discharged as labor begins and the cervix begins to dilate in preparation of delivery of the fetus.

In addition to the fetus, the uterus also contains a developing organ called the placenta, the organ through which the fetus receives nourishment and to which the fetus is connected by the umbilical cord.

- A sac of amniotic fluid (bag of waters) surrounds the fetus while in utero to cushion and protect the fetus. This sac will usually rupture on its own (often the precursor of active labor).

- Occasionally the sac will deliver unruptured with the baby and must be torn by the EMT to allow the baby to breathe.
- Crowning is when the baby's head is visible in the birth canal.

The perineum is the area between a female's vagina and anus. This is commonly torn during the delivery of a fetus. In a hospital setting, an obstetrician or midwife may cut this area before crowning to expedite delivery. This procedure is called an episiotomy; the perineum is then stitched after birth to facilitate healing.

Labor

Labor is the process of delivery of a fetus and is defined as beginning with the first pronounced uterine contraction and terminating with the delivery of the placenta. It is subdivided into three stages:

- The first stage of labor occurs as contractions begin and may last from a few minutes to many hours. The contractions can be palpated on the mother's abdomen. These contractions cause the cervix to dilate in preparation for the baby's expulsion from the uterus.
- The second stage of labor is reached when the cervix is fully dilated and the baby's head begins to enter the birth canal. It is at this stage that the EMT should be able to observe the baby's head during the contraction. This stage culminates with the delivery of the baby.
- The third stage of labor is the delivery of the placenta.

The first part of the baby that is visible is referred to as the *presenting part* and usually will be the baby's head. If any other part of the baby presents first, this is referred to as a *breech delivery*.

Each EMS unit should carry an obstetrical kit, ideally at least two. These kits may be pre-assembled, or standard prepackaged kits may be purchased. Each kit, at minimum, should include:

- Surgical scissors or scalpel
- Two hemostats or cord clamps
- A bulb syringe
- Sterile towels
- 2 × 10 gauze sponges
- Sterile gloves
- A sterile baby blanket
- Sanitary napkins
- Biohazard plastic bag

Obstetrical Assessment

Assessment of a patient in labor is the same as any other medical assessment, but with several additions. It is useful to know which pregnancy this is for the mother. A first pregnancy will usually have a longer labor period than a fourth or fifth pregnancy.

Document a patient in labor as follows:

- **Para** is the number of live births the mother has had.
- **Gravida** is the number of times the mother has been pregnant.
- If a woman has been pregnant three times, with two miscarriages and one live birth, it would be written as **P1 G3**.

While this may be considered private or uncomfortable information for the EMT to ask, the patient or a bystander should also be asked if her prior pregnancies have ended in live births or miscarriages, whether the live births were vaginal deliveries or Caesarean sections, and whether there were any specific complications with her prior births. Some women may deny that they are pregnant due to social stigma or other concerns, and you may have to rely on your own observations about whether an obstetrical emergency exists. If the patient is in active labor, you must ask how far apart the contractions are and how long they last. The longer the contractions and the more frequently they occur, the more likely that delivery is imminent.

Miscarriage/Abortion

The EMT must be aware of the predelivery emergency conditions that may be encountered. The first is spontaneous abortion or miscarriage. A miscarriage is when the products of conception are delivered early in the pregnancy. This will usually be dispatched as "female vaginal bleeding" or "female hemorrhaging." The assessment and care of the patient will be the same as for any patient with severe hemorrhaging. If the products of conception are available, they should be placed in a plastic bag and transported to the hospital out of the sight of the mother for the obstetrician to evaluate.

A miscarriage is an emotionally traumatic event for both the mother and the family, and prehospital care for the emotional trauma is as important as the physical care. The EMT must be supportive and encouraging, just as he or she would be if a patient's loved one had died. The pain of loss should not be minimized by the EMT because the loss is not a fully developed human being. Statements like "You can always have another child" are minimizing statements and may not even be true. Support is often best given by conveying your concern and sense of loss to the mother.

Some women may also elect to have a scheduled medical abortion, which may involve a process called a dilation and curettage (D&C), a procedure to remove tissue from inside the uterus. This can lead to hemorrhaging directly after or for a few days after the procedure has been done. There are also times when a woman may not have had a sterile procedure done, in which case there may be internal damage that requires bleeding control as well as infection worries to consider. Regardless of how the procedure was done, there is often abdominal pain or tenderness after the procedure and EMS may be summoned. It is not up to the EMT to judge a woman's decision to have an abortion, no matter their own personal beliefs. The EMT is there to provide appropriate medical care and delivery to the proper medical facility.

In the case of hypovolemic shock or low blood volume due to hemorrhage, the EMT must be prepared for an expedited transport or to call ALS for backup, if they are closer than a facility is. Shock management includes keeping the patient warm, providing oxygen, managing the bleeding, and constantly assessing vital signs.

Keep in mind there may also be a need for psychological support. Regardless of why or how the mother has lost a child, it is still a loss or upsetting situation for the female patient. Be empathetic and document as factually as possible. Be an advocate for your patient always.

Complications in Pregnancy

While many pregnancies are smooth and uncomplicated, some women experience complications that develop acutely or slowly over time.

Table 6.16 *Pregnancy Complications*

Complication	Key Ideas
Ectopic Pregnancy	• **Egg is fertilized outside the uterus** • Most commonly these fertilizations happen in the fallopian tubes, but rarely they may also happen in the abdominal tissue • Are nonviable, meaning that they will not result in a live birth • Bleeding from ectopic pregnancy causes 10% of all pregnancy-related deaths, and it's the leading cause of first-trimester maternal death • If the patient was hopeful for a pregnancy, there is an element of psychological support that will need to be provided as well
Seizure (medical emergency, regardless of the cause)	• Has various causes, i.e., hypoglycemia, epilepsy, anoxia, and eclampsia; a thorough assessment should identify the underlying reason • Transport patient left lateral recumbent to allow for the best possible blood flow and avoid constricting the inferior vena cava

Pre-eclampsia & Eclampsia	• **Characterized by high blood pressure and signs of damage to another organ system; if untreated, can result in seizures**
	• Usually begins after 20 weeks of pregnancy in women whose blood pressure had been normal (below 140/90)
	• Hypertension may develop slowly over time, or it may have a sudden onset
	• Sudden weight gain and edema, particularly in face and hands, can be an early indicator but is not always accurate
	• Other symptoms can include:
	  – Severe headache
	  – Nausea and vomiting
	  – Shortness of breath
	  – Decreased urine output and excess protein in urine
	  – Upper abdominal pain

(Continued)

Table 6.16 *Pregnancy Complications (Continued)*

Complication	Key Ideas
Supine Hypotensive Syndrome	• **Compression of the inferior vena cava and aorta by the fetus leading to decreased venous return and resulting hypoperfusion in the supine (upward) position** • Loss of consciousness and even maternal and/or fetal death can occur • Symptoms (typically seen 3–10 minutes after lying down) can include: 　– Tachycardia 　– Diaphoresis 　– Nausea/vomiting 　– Weakness/dizziness/light-headedness 　– Pallor
Abruptio Placenta	• **Partial or complete separation of the placenta from the inner wall of the uterus before delivery** • Can decrease or block the baby's supply of oxygen and nutrients • Causes heavy bleeding in the mother—internally and/or externally • Symptoms include abdominal and back pain • Most likely to occur in the last trimester of pregnancy, often closer to the due date
Placenta Previa	• **Placenta lies lower in the uterus than the usual position and partially or completely covers the cervix** • Typically occurs in the third trimester • More common in women who have had multiple births or a previous cesarean section (C-section) birth • Most common symptom is painless vaginal bleeding; premature contractions may occur • If diagnosed, typical treatment is bedrest for the mother
Vaginal Bleeding (serious, regardless of whether accompanied by abdominal pain)	• Can be controlled by application of sanitary napkins to the external vagina • Manage shock symptoms if present • Transport should be expedited if bleeding is heavy or uncontrolled
Traumatic Injury	• Treat like any other trauma victim, with special attention to the abdomen and vagina for signs of bleeding • If spinal immobilization is indicated, place the patient on spine board, with pillows underneath the right side so board tilts to the left; if spinal immobilization is not indicated, transport the patient on her left side • Remember that you have 2 patients, the mother and the child, so reassess frequently

Emergency Procedures for Delivery

If the call is for a normal first-stage labor patient and delivery does not appear to be imminent based upon the primary assessment, then the EMT must complete the secondary assessment and determine if there is enough time to transport the patient safely to the hospital or if it would be safer to deliver the baby at the current location. This decision should be made in consultation with medical control, which will want to know specific symptoms and vital signs.

If the baby is crowning and delivery is imminent, the EMT should open the emergency obstetrics kit and prepare for delivery. Proper BSI precautions include sterile gloves, mask, gown, and eye protection. The procedures are as follows:

- The mother should lie on her back in a semi-Fowler position, propped up with pillows and with her knees drawn up and spread apart. Elevate the mother's buttocks with blankets or pillows.

- Create a sterile field around the vagina using paper barriers or towels. Do not touch the mother's vagina except during delivery if necessary to maintain the baby's airway, and even then, only when your partner is present.

- As the baby's head is delivered, apply gentle pressure on the skull to prevent explosive delivery, avoiding the baby's fontanelle, or soft spot.

- If the amniotic sac is still intact, puncture it and pull it away from the baby's mouth and nose as they appear.

- As the baby's head is delivered, check that the cord is not wrapped around the neck (**nuchal cord**). If it is, try and unwrap it. If that is not possible, clamp the cord and cut it between the clamps.

- After the head is delivered, support the head with one hand and suction the mouth and nose two or three times with the bulb syringe. Turn the baby so the shoulders are horizontal instead of vertical, as this will help facilitate the rest of the body sliding out. The torso and the rest of the body will usually be delivered with the next contraction. As the feet are delivered, grab the feet with one hand and wipe the blood and mucus from the mouth and nose with sterile gauze.

- If the baby is breathing normally, wrap the baby in a warm blanket, being sure to cover the baby's head to minimize heat loss. Place the baby on its side, the head slightly lower than the trunk. The baby should be level with the mother's vagina until the cord is cut.

- With the baby stable, and if the cord was not wrapped around the neck and cut already, clamp the cord 3–4 inches from the baby and cut the cord between the clamps once the pulsations of the cord have ceased.

- If the baby and the mother are stable, the EMT should prepare to deliver the placenta. As the uterus contracts, the EMT should urge the mother to push and expel the placenta. Once the placenta is delivered, place the placenta in the plastic bag and transport it along with the baby and mother to the hospital. The obstetrician will want to examine the placenta to be sure that all of it was expelled.

- Place two sanitary napkins over the vagina and have the mother close her legs. Have the mother massage her uterus through her abdomen to assist in the control of bleeding.
- If the mother begins to exhibit signs of shock (pale and diaphoretic), administer oxygen via non-rebreather and expedite transport.

APGAR Score

Patient assessment of a neonate (newborn baby) includes the APGAR score, which should be performed at 1 minute postpartum and 5 minutes postpartum. This index gives an excellent overall summary of the baby's condition and will alert the receiving hospital to the actual condition. APGAR stands for *Appearance, Pulse, Grimace, Activity,* and *Respirations.*

It is a good idea to have this scorecard posted on the action wall of the truck. Each item receives 0, 1, or 2 points. The maximum score is 10 points, and the minimum is 0.

Sign	0 Points	1 Point	2 Points
Appearance	Baby is cyanotic or pale	Baby's torso is pink, but extremities are bluish	Baby's extremities are pink
Pulse	No pulse	Heart rate <100 per min	Heart rate >100 per min
Grimace (tested by flicking baby's feet)	No response	Slight facial grimace	Baby grimaces, coughs, sneezes, or cries
Activity	No movement/limp	Some flexion of extremities	Baby is actively moving
Respiration	No respiration	Slow and irregular breathing/weak cry	Good respiration/strong cry

The number of personnel available may dictate that this assessment not be done; for example, a finding of no respirations should lead the EMT to begin respiratory assistance and not to spend time recording assessment findings.

APGAR scoring is as follows:

- **7–10 points**: neonate is in good condition.
- **4–6 points**: neonate is moderately depressed, and stimulation and oxygen are indicated.
- **0–3 points**: neonate requires aggressive resuscitation, including positive ventilation and chest compressions.

Abnormal Delivery

Abnormal delivery situations are rare, but still are a concern to the EMT. Some situations requiring EMT intervention are as follows:

- **Prolapsed cord** is a condition in which the cord presents from the vagina before the head of the baby is delivered. This presents a serious emergency for the viability of the fetus. Treatment for this condition, in addition to normal assessment and oxygenation for the mother, includes placing the mother's head below her buttocks to lessen pressure on the birth canal and fetus. If the cord is still pulsating, insert a gloved hand into the vagina and push the presenting part of the fetus away from the cord to prevent the pressure of the neonate from cutting off the flow of blood through the cord. Transport immediately and continue to monitor the pulsation of the cord.

- **Breech presentation** is where any part of the fetus other than the head presents through the birth canal first. This requires immediate transport upon recognition. The mother should be placed on high-flow oxygen and transported in a head down position with her pelvis elevated.

- **Meconium aspiration** occurs when a neonate, due to distress during labor, defecates into the amniotic fluid and then aspirates this fluid as it begins to breathe. The presence of meconium is detectable when the amniotic fluid is greenish or yellowish brown instead of clear. If meconium is detected, the EMT should aspirate the oropharynx before trying to stimulate spontaneous respirations.

- **Premature birth**, i.e., before the full 37-week gestation period, poses an especially high risk of hypothermia to infants; the babies must be kept warm (especially the crown of the head) so they can retain heat. Early premature infants—less than 30 weeks—will also usually require manual resuscitation.

Gynecological Emergencies

Gynecological emergencies also present special considerations, especially for male EMTs who may be sensitive or embarrassed by treating female genitalia. Severe vaginal bleeding is treated in the same way as any other internal hemorrhage, with oxygen and immediate transport.

Special sensitivity is required in dealing with women who have been sexually assaulted. It is always preferable to have a female EMT be the primary caregiver if possible, as the victim may be fearful of any male at this time, especially those in uniform who are projecting an image of power.

- The primary EMT should take a thoughtful, nonjudgmental approach with victims of sexual assault. The key words are sensitivity, support, and professionalism.

- Aside from taking the normal trauma assessment protocols, preserve all evidence for possible criminal prosecution.

- Discourage the patient from showering, bathing, or voiding, if possible.

- A good practice is to fully open the stretcher bed sheet and allow the patient to wrap themselves if wanted. This can provide a "cocoon" feeling, which may not only make them feel safe and enclosed but also allow any blood, hair, etc., to collect on the sheet, as the hospital or police offers may use it as more evidence.

- Visual examination of the genitalia should be conducted only if profuse bleeding is present.

- Depending on your state, as a medical practitioner you may be required to report any sexual assault that you learn has occurred.

Practice Set

1. Which of the following medications can cause hypotension?

   A. Nitroglycerin

   B. Aspirin

   C. Oxygen

   D. Epinephrine

2. What is the dosage for nitroglycerin in the spray or tablet form?

   A. 0.2 mg

   B. 1 mg

   C. 4 mg

   D. 0.4 mg

3. Which of the following is the correct dosage and administration route of epinephrine for an adult to be delivered by EMTs?

   A. 0.15 mg; IM

   B. 0.15 mg; IN

   C. 0.3 mg; IM

   D. 0.3 mg; IN

4. You respond to a call for difficulty breathing. Arriving on scene, you find a male in his sixties breathing rapidly and sitting in tripod position. His color is bluish, and he is sweaty and cool to the touch. You perform your initial assessment, which is unremarkable, and his vital signs are all within normal range except for his respiratory rate, which is 22. What is your first medication of choice to treat this patient?

   A. Epinephrine

   B. Albuterol

   C. Nitroglycerin

   D. Oxygen

5. In the scenario in question 4, what device, dosage, and route would you use to administer the drug?

   A. 0.3 mg epinephrine via subcutaneous injection

   B. 2 liters per minute oxygen via nasal cannula

   C. 12 liters per minute oxygen via non-rebreather mask

   D. 1 puff albuterol via metered inhaler

6. Which of the following signs and symptoms is indicative of inadequate air exchange?

   A. Breath sounds clear in all fields

   B. Chest rises and falls with each breath

   C. Respiratory rate between 12 and 20 times per minute

   D. Altered mental status

7. You arrive on the scene of a call for difficulty breathing. You enter the kitchen and you see a 70-year-old male seated at the table leaning forward. He is having severe trouble breathing, his skin is bluish-gray, and he is sweaty. You hear a gurgling sound as he tries to inhale. As you ask him questions, he tries to respond between gasps, but his answers are not comprehensible. He is clutching his chest and appears to be in severe pain. His wife advises you that he had a heart attack last year and takes nitroglycerin, hydrochlorothiazide, and digitalis. The chest pains began as he finished supper. The patient took two NTG tablets, but the pain has continued to get worse. His vital signs are BP 180/120, pulse 120, respiratory rate 28, pulse oximetry 82%. What is your next intervention?

   A. Load and go

   B. Oxygen 15 lpm via non-rebreather

   C. Contact medical control for NTG 0.4 mg

   D. Apply the AED and analyze his cardiac rhythm

8. You have made the load-and-go decision on the patient in question 7 and removed him immediately to the truck after you've applied the oxygen mask at high flow. As you begin your focused exam en route to the hospital, you notice your patient is now unconscious and has stopped breathing, and you cannot palpate a carotid pulse. You instruct your partner to begin ventilating the patient with a BVM and OPA and hook up the AED to the patient. You ask the driver to stop while you analyze the patient with the AED. The AED reads "no shock advised." Which of the following statements is correct as your next action?

   A. Deliver two breaths using BVM, then start compressions

   B. Contact medical control for permission to administer NTG 0.4 mg sublingually

   C. Continue transport with no further intervention

   D. Begin chest compressions for 2 minutes and then reanalyze with the AED

9. You are dispatched to a call for a man down. You arrive on scene and find a male in his seventies lying on his back on the front lawn. There are no bystanders or family members present. He is cyanotic, pulseless, and apneic. He is cool to the touch, and when you try to move his limbs and jaw, they are rigid and do not move. You pull his shirt up and notice that the anterior portion of his torso is pale and the posterior is black-and-blue, with a definitive line between the two areas. Which of the following conditions should you suspect?

   A. Cardiac arrest

   B. Myocardial infarction

   C. Apnea secondary to COPD

   D. Biological death

10. You are dispatched to a residence for a male patient with a possible myocardial infarction. Prior to administering him nitroglycerin, which of the following medications should you ask the patient if he has taken?

    A. Tylenol™

    B. Lasix™

    C. Viagra™

    D. Prilosec™

11. Which of the following best describes the condition atherosclerosis?

    A. Hardening of the arteries

    B. Chest pain that goes away with rest

    C. Buildup of plaque in the arteries

    D. Plaque that traveled to the brain

12. You are dispatched to the front lawn of a residence for a possible heart attack. You respond emergently and arrive on scene wearing the proper protective equipment. The scene is safe, and you see a male in his mid-eighties lying supine on the lawn. He appears unresponsive and cyanotic with his mouth and eyes open. You perform an airway maneuver, and he has no spontaneous respirations; you cannot detect a carotid pulse. What is your next procedure?

    A. Ask bystanders to call 911

    B. Request an ALS intercept

    C. Perform CPR

    D. Administer 325 mg aspirin PO

13. Ventricular fibrillation is a condition affecting which system of the heart?

    A. Electrical

    B. Circulatory

    C. Mechanical

    D. All of the above

14. Which is the proper procedure for correction of the condition in question 13 by an EMT?

    A. Use a BVM to deliver breaths

    B. Shock by AED

    C. Call ALS

    D. CPR

15. You arrive on the scene of an unknown medical call to a residence. The husband advises that he went to check on his wife and found her unresponsive. He directs you to the bedroom, where there is a female lying supine, pale, and cyanotic in bed. She does not appear to be breathing and has no carotid pulse. What must you do before beginning CPR?

    A. Call Medical Control

    B. Place her on a hard surface

    C. Hook up your AED and shock as advised

    D. Request an ALS intercept

16. You are dispatched to a college dorm room for a report of a man down. You respond emergently and arrive on scene with suitable protective equipment and have determined that the scene is safe. You find an 18-year-old male lying on his back, unconscious and not responsive to any stimuli. He has an airway and is making snoring sounds at a regular rate. As you are checking his breathing, you notice that his breath has a fruity odor. His carotid pulse is strong, rapid, and regular. His girlfriend is also in the room and is hysterical as she tells you they were sitting talking when he suddenly collapsed. What question do you want to ask the girlfriend next?

    A. "Does he have any allergies?"

    B. "Is he diabetic?"

    C. "Is this a frequent occurrence?"

    D. "Does he take any medications on a regular basis?"

17. What type of stroke is caused by a burst vessel in the brain, which causes bleeding?

    A. TIA

    B. Infarction

    C. Hemorrhagic

    D. Ischemic

18. Which of the following conditions may cause a seizure?

    A. High body temperature

    B. Head injury

    C. Epilepsy

    D. All of the above

19. The most important procedure for an EMT to perform in dealing with a seizure patient is to

    A. secure the airway.

    B. secure the patient's limbs with restraints.

    C. administer oral glucose.

    D. transport priority.

20. You are dispatched to a restaurant for a report of difficulty breathing. You respond emergently wearing appropriate protective equipment, and there are no scene safety concerns. You are directed to a table where a male and a female are seated. The female has her hand to her throat and appears to be in respiratory distress. She is moving air with difficulty, and her male companion is upset. She is unable to answer your questions, and her companion knows of no medical history, medications, or allergies. He advises that she had just eaten a shrimp cocktail when the symptoms suddenly developed. The patient is pale and diaphoretic, with a rapid pulse. The police officer who searched her pocketbook for her driver's license hands you an EpiPen™ that he found in the pocketbook. What should you do at this point?

    A. Administer the EpiPen™ to the lateral thigh

    B. Have your partner call medical control while you prepare to ventilate the patient

    C. Administer oxygen via nasal cannula at 10 liters per minute

    D. Place the patient on a stretcher and transport priority to the nearest medical facility

21. You are on duty in your station when a male subject comes running in. He is pale, diaphoretic, and short of breath. He keeps stammering the word "bee" and is pointing to his arm, where you notice a large welt. He is unable to respond to your questions and is beginning to lose consciousness. What condition do you suspect?

    A. Anaphylaxis

    B. Diabetes

    C. Myocardial infarction

    D. Epilepsy

22. You are dispatched to a residence for a possible overdose. You arrive on the scene and find police have secured the area. You are wearing appropriate protective apparel. The husband advises that his wife has been despondent and he fears she may have overdosed on her prescription tranquilizers. He states that she has been drinking all day and is now semiconscious. In the bedroom, you find a female in her fifties who appears to be sleeping. She is supine, making snoring sounds, and has a slow pulse. She responds when you call her name but will not answer any questions. Her gaze is unfocused, and her pupils are dilated and do not respond to light. There is an empty bottle of Clonazepam™ next to the bed that was refilled yesterday and contained 30 one mg tablets. There is also an empty fifth of gin, and her breath smells of alcohol. Her husband states that she entered the bedroom 15 minutes before he called 911. Her vital signs are 100/60, respirations 12, and pulse 55. What is your next course of action?

    A. Transport

    B. Contact medical control

    C. Administer 0.2 mg Naloxone IN

    D. Administer 50 mg of activated charcoal

23. You are dispatched to meet the police at a residence with no other information available. You arrive on scene and police lead you to a subject seated in his car, which is parked in his garage. The officer tells you that when they arrived, the garage door was closed and the car was running. Police have shut the engine off and left the doors open. You enter the garage and observe a male seated behind the wheel of a car. He is unconscious and not responding to any stimuli. He is cyanotic, with slow, shallow respirations and a weak, thready pulse. What should you suspect as the cause of his unconsciousness?

    A. Heart attack

    B. Seizure

    C. Stroke

    D. Carbon-monoxide poisoning

24. In the scenario in question 23, as you arrive and meet with the police officer, what determination should you have initially made with the information he has given you?

    A. This is a load and go.

    B. This is a crime scene that must be preserved.

    C. The scene is unsafe.

    D. This call needs an advanced life support unit.

25. In the scenario in question 23, you find the victim has been extricated to the front lawn by police prior to EMS arrival. You have performed your assessments, and the vital signs are blood pressure 110/80, pulse 50, respirations 12 and shallow. Pulse oximeter shows that his oxygen saturation is 98%. What should be your next intervention?

    A. Do nothing

    B. Administer 15 lpm oxygen

    C. ALS

    D. Administer 6 lpm via nasal cannula

26. In the scenario in question 25, which piece of specialized equipment might influence your choice of destination hospital?

    A. Heart-lung machine

    B. Hyperbaric chamber

    C. CPAP machine

    D. Positive pressure ventilators

27. What body temperature is considered to be moderately hypothermic?

    A. 81°F

    B. 91°F

    C. 93°F

    D. 89°F

28. You arrive on the scene of a motor vehicle accident on a cold snowy evening. The outside temperature is 0°F. You observe a subject lying in the snow next to a wrecked car. Police are on scene, and you are wearing appropriate protective gear. The patient is a 35-year-old male, semiconscious, breathing rapidly and with a weak, thready pulse. You detect the odor of alcohol on his breath. As you palpate his torso, beneath his shirt you notice he is cold to the touch, but is not shivering. His hands and feet feel cold and rigid. Which stage of hypothermia do you suspect?

    A. Mild stage

    B. Moderate stage

    C. Severe stage

    D. Frostbite stage

29. In the scenario in question 28, you find two additional patients who have been ejected from the car and who present the same symptoms. One is a 78-year-old female, and the other is a 32-year-old female. Which of the following should be treated first?

    A. 35-year-old male

    B. 78-year-old female

    C. 32-year-old female

    D. Treatment should occur at the receiving facility.

30. In the scenario in question 29, you have removed the 78-year-old female to your truck and have begun transport. In addition to her lethargy, her vital signs are beginning to drop. You notice that her right hand was not gloved and now appears whitish and waxy. Which of the following treatments would be appropriate for this patient?

    A. Warm packs under her arms, beneath her neck, and between her legs

    B. Warm water bath for her right hand

    C. Oxygen

    D. All of the above

31. You are standing by a summer road race and are summoned to a runner who has fallen. The patient is an 18-year-old female who is lying underneath a tree, clutching her right leg. She is breathing rapidly and is flushed. Her skin is hot and dry. Which of the following conditions do you suspect and should you treat first?

    A. Heat cramps

    B. Heat exhaustion

    C. Heatstroke

    D. Heat conduction

32. You are en route back to the station from the hospital when you observe a subject in the water 30 feet from a lake shore and appearing to be in distress. You notify your dispatcher and stand on the shore. The subject is flailing his arms and yelling, "Help!" Your own swimming ability is limited, and your partner cannot swim at all. What should be your next course of action?

    A. Dive in, swimming to the victim as quickly as possible

    B. Attempt to throw him the rescue rope from the truck

    C. Drive back to the station and get a boat

    D. Buddy-swim with your partner to the victim

33. You are dispatched to a residence for an unknown-type medical call. An adult female tells you she was working in her garden when she felt a stinging sensation on the back of her left arm. She is conscious, alert, and oriented times three with normal respirations and pulse. She has no significant medical history and no known allergies. You examine her left arm and see a bright red area 5 inches in diameter with a white spot in the center and a small black speck in the center of the white spot. What is your next course of action?

    A. Contact medical control

    B. Administer epinephrine via auto-injector

    C. Scrape the black speck off with a credit card

    D. Administer oxygen 10 liters per minute via non-rebreather mask

34. You are dispatched to a residence for a woman in labor. You arrive on scene, having taken the usual precautions, and observe a female in her early thirties lying on the couch in the living room. She advises you that this is her third pregnancy, her bag of waters ruptured 30 minutes ago, and her pains are increasing in intensity and are currently 3 minutes apart. Which of the following should be your next move?

    A. Place her on the stretcher and respond emergently to the nearest maternity unit

    B. Tie her legs together to prevent premature birth and expedite transport

    C. Remove her underwear and at the next contraction, examine the birth canal for signs of crowning

    D. Insert your hand into the birth canal and see if you can feel the baby's head

35. In the scenario in question 34, you take vital signs and prepare for transport. The mother suddenly tells you she is having a contraction, and you observe the top of the baby's head as her labia separate. What should you now do?

    A. Place her on the stretcher and respond emergently to the nearest maternity unit

    B. Open the obstetrical kit and prepare for delivery

    C. Administer 15 lpm oxygen to the mother

    D. Call ALS, as this is a higher-level call

36. In the scenario in question 34, instead of the top of the baby's head, you see the baby's arm protruding from the mother's vagina. What should you now prepare to do?

    A. Place her on the stretcher and respond emergently to the nearest hospital that has maternity capabilities

    B. Open the obstetrical kit and prepare for delivery

    C. Pull gently on the arm to facilitate delivery

    D. Wait for the next contraction and see if the condition rectifies itself

37. You are dispatched along with police to an unknown-type medical call. You arrive simultaneously with the police and observe a large male trying to throw a refrigerator at his wife. You assist police in wrestling the man to a prone position, and the police handcuff his wrists behind his back as he continues to struggle and curse. His wife advises you that he has no medical problems, takes no medication, and has no history of any psychological problems. She indicates he was behaving normally until she asked if he would like a cup of tea, at which point he suddenly assaulted her and became violent. The police place him under arrest and try to place him in a squad car. What is your role as the medical provider?

    A. Assist the police in subduing and arresting the subject

    B. Intervene and insist that he be transported via ambulance to the hospital

    C. Go back in service as this is a police matter

    D. Remove his restraints, place him on your stretcher, and transport

38. In the scenario in question 37, how should this patient be restrained by EMS?

    A. Leave him in handcuffs and use leg irons to secure his ankles to his wrists in a prone position

    B. Place him in a supine position on a backboard and secure his limbs with soft restraints

    C. Place him a supine position on a backboard with his hands cuffed behind his back, place another backboard on top of him, and secure the backboards together with handcuffs

    D. Remove his metal restraints, wrap him in a blanket, and secure him to the stretcher with soft restraints

39. You are dispatched to a college dorm for a possible diabetic emergency. You respond emergently and arrive on scene. As you walk down the hallway, you observe a female whom you have previously treated for hypoglycemia secondary to diabetes talking and humming to herself. She is walking near the edge of a high balcony. Her roommates tell you that she has been behaving strangely all morning. What should be your next move?

    A. Tackle her and restrain her

    B. Administer 15 mg oral glucose

    C. Request police assistance

    D. Take her by the arm and gently sit her in a chair for a more thorough evaluation

40. In the scenario in question 39, your evaluation reveals that the patient's answers are incoherent and inappropriate, her blood pressure is 120/80, her pulse is 72, and her respirations are 12. Her blood glucose is 76. She does not refuse to be transported and allows you to lead her to the truck, where you place her in a semi-Fowler position and secure her to the stretcher with the normal straps. She now tries to unfasten the straps and pushes your arm away. What should you do?

    A. Restrain her arms with soft restraints

    B. Handcuff her hands to the middle strap

    C. Call for police backup

    D. Contact medical control for permission to restrain

Answers and Explanations

1. A

Nitroglycerin can cause hypotension because it causes the vessels to vasodilate (open).

2. D

Please refer back to the pharmacology section and table if unsure.

3. C

IM stands for intramuscular while IN stands for intranasal. 0.15 mg is the pediatric dosage for epinephrine, while 0.3 mg is the adult dosage. Epinephrine is delivered IM on the mid-lateral thigh, most commonly through an auto-injector pen.

4. D

This patient is presenting signs of hypoxia, and almost all state protocols allow the EMT to administer oxygen for immediate relief. Epinephrine is indicated for an allergic reaction, albuterol for airway obstruction, and nitroglycerin for chest pain. Albuterol may be indicated if the dyspnea is being caused by constricted bronchioles, but permission must first be obtained from medical control following a detailed assessment. Oxygen is always the first drug of choice in these situations.

5. C

The patient's condition requires high-flow oxygen (10–15 liters per minute), and the correct device to deliver this flow is the non-rebreather mask. Epinephrine is indicated for anaphylaxis, low-flow oxygen (2 lpm) would be indicated for mild hypoxia or dyspnea, and a metered inhaler for difficulty breathing caused by airway obstruction.

6. D

(A), (B), and (C) are all indicative of normal respiratory pattern. Altered mental status may be caused by insufficient oxygen supply to the brain.

7. B

This patient is having severe difficulty breathing, and his pulse oximetry and skin color indicate hypoxia. This is a moderately difficult question, as all of the other answers could also be considered correct actions over the course of time. However, the question asks what your next course of action is, and this would be to try and relieve the hypoxia with supplemental oxygen therapy.

8. D

The current protocols require chest compressions before breaths, in the C-A-B sequence. (B) is incorrect because the patient's problem at this time has progressed from chest pain to cardiac arrest. (C) also is incorrect, as protocols require CPR for this patient until ordered to discontinue by a physician.

9. D

This patient exhibits the signs and symptoms of rigor mortis and postmortem lividity, which will allow you in most jurisdictions to not perform CPR and turn this case over to law enforcement for investigation of sudden death. The cause of the sudden death may have been any of the other answers.

10. C

It is important to ask the patient if he has taken Viagra™ (sildenafil citrate) within the last 24 hours. If he has, nitroglycerin is contraindicated because it can cause a sudden and severe drop in blood pressure.

11. C

Hardening of the arteries (A) is often the result of atherosclerosis, but they are two separate conditions. (B) describes angina, while (D) describes what can happen during a stroke.

12. C

The correct action is to perform CPR. (A) is incorrect, since somebody has already called 911 and you are on scene. You should have requested the ALS intercept when dispatched to the possible heart call. Aspirin is indicated for chest pain, but this patient is unconscious and unresponsive and should not be given anything by mouth.

13. D

Ventricular fibrillation occurs when the electrical system of the heart no longer energizes the heart to pump properly and instead just vibrates (fibrillates) the cardiac muscle. (D) is correct because while it is an electrical problem overall, if the electricity is out, then the pump (the heart) will stop working (mechanical) and then circulation stops as well. Ventricular fibrillation is considered a lethal rhythm and needs to be corrected by an electrical charge (AED or manual defibrillation).

14. B

Shock by AED is the correct answer. (A), (C), and (D) are indicated, but should not delay in providing the AED shock.

15. B

The chest compressions of CPR are the most effective if the patient is lying on a hard, flat surface. CPR done on a mattress is not as effective, since there is not enough pressure created in the thoracic cavity to compress the heart and initiate the pumping action. It is not necessary for an EMT to contact Medical Control to begin CPR. An ALS intercept should be requested, but not at the expense of time for beginning CPR.

16. B

You should consider diabetes because of the fruity odor of this patient's breath, which could be indicative of hypoglycemia. The key word in the question is "next." It is always important to fully read each question and each answer and find the one that is *most* appropriate.

17. C

The correct answer is (C), with the key word being hemorrhage, which means bleeding. Infarction is typically referred to when speaking of a heart attack, not a stroke, but is the body's reaction to a lack of perfusion. This closely relates to ischemia, which can be caused by a blockage in a vessel, which describes (D).

18. D

Any of the answers may cause a seizure.

19. A

If you are answering an exam question that describes a medical emergency, you cannot forget the basics. You must identify the most important procedure (and the focus of the EMT's attention in any given emergency)—maintaining a patent airway. Securing the patient's limbs (B) may be a secondary consideration, and a priority transport (D) is probably indicated but not the most important. (C) is not indicated, despite hypoglycemia being a possible cause of seizures.

20. A

The EMT does not need to contact medical control to administer the EpiPen™ according to the National Scope of Practice. Supplemental oxygen will help the hypoxia, but needs to be given by non-rebreather mask at 10–15 lpm. Also, quick transport may not be sufficient if the airway is closing quickly. This patient is suffering an acute allergic reaction to shellfish and needs epinephrine immediately.

21. A

The patient is probably having an allergic (anaphylactic) reaction to a bee sting, as evidenced by his symptoms and his repeating the word "bee." A diabetic emergency would cause him to lose consciousness, a myocardial infarction (heart attack) is usually accompanied by chest pains, and epilepsy is a condition that causes seizures followed by loss of consciousness.

22. A

This patient should be transported immediately. (B) should be done while en route. (C) is used for opioid drugs, which Clonazepam is not; it is also not the correct dosage. (D) may be indicated in some systems, but is not indicated on a national level in the scope of practice for EMTs.

23. D

Circumstances would indicate that a running car in a closed garage emitting carbon monoxide, a poison, has caused this condition, although the others cannot be ruled out initially.

24. C

EMS personnel should not enter this environment without proper respiratory protection, such as a self-contained breathing apparatus. To do so invites possible carbon-monoxide poisoning, which delays proper care to the initial patient and complicates the entire rescue by adding to the total number of victims who must be treated. (A) and (B) might be correct if the scene were safe. Regarding (D), there is nothing in this scenario that would indicate the intervention of an ALS unit.

25. B

This patient is severely hypoxic as indicated by his physical appearance, and high-flow oxygen therapy is indicated. The high pulse oximeter is grossly misleading in carbon-monoxide poisoning, as it can give a false high reading due to the presence of carbon monoxide in the red blood cells, and thus cannot be relied on in this case.

26. B

The hyperbaric chamber, in which outside oxygen pressure is increased, has proven effective in treatment of carbon-monoxide poisoning. This decision may be made by protocol or medical control, but if you are given the choice between two hospital emergency departments, go with the hospital that has the hyperbaric chamber. (A) is normal equipment for any hospital with a full operating suite and would not be necessary for treating carbon-monoxide poisoning. (D) is standard equipment in any hospital emergency department, and (C) is located in most ambulances as a piece of standard equipment.

27. D

Moderate hypothermia is between 82–90°F, which makes all the other answers incorrect, except for (D).

28. C

The absence of shivering means the patient has moved beyond the mild stage. Moderate hypothermia is marked by increasing mental apathy and loss of motor function, but severe stage is when the extremities begin to freeze. While frostbite is present in the severe stage, it is only a symptom, not a whole stage of events, so the correct answer is (C).

29. B

The elderly person is more at risk for increasing hypothermia due to her age.

30. D

The patient is in fourth-stage hypothermia and needs to be warmed. In addition, she has symptoms of frostbite to her right hand that can be treated en route with a warm water bath. Oxygen is indicated for this patient due to her increasing lethargy.

31. C

While (A) and (B) may seem correct, in reading the question you must be able to identify that heatstroke is the most serious of the three and the condition you should be concerned about. This patient has a high core temperature and her body's heat-regulating mechanisms are not working, so she must be cooled down with cold packs to the axillary, cervical, and groin areas.

32. B

Never undertake a rescue unless you are confident in your abilities to perform the necessary activity. Since neither you nor your partner is trained in water rescue techniques, you should not attempt to swim to the patient. If you have an object to throw to the victim, this is your best course of action. Leaving the scene to go and get a boat could be considered abandonment of the patient. Since your partner cannot swim, a buddy swim is not a possibility, nor does it solve the problem of being able to approach and assist the victim.

33. C

The patient's symptoms are consistent with a bee sting, and she is giving no evidence at this time of anaphylaxis. You should, however, continue to monitor the patient and urge her to go to the emergency department for a more definitive diagnosis.

34. C

The correct next step is to look for crowning. (A) is incorrect, since you have not yet performed an adequate assessment. (B) is never correct, as it will endanger both the baby and the mother. (D) is also incorrect, since the only time you place your gloved hand into the birth canal is to assist in maintaining the baby's airway or to loosen the cord if it is wrapped around the baby's neck.

35. B

The correct next action is to prepare for delivery. (A) is incorrect, since with the baby crowning delivery is now imminent, and you are probably better off in the living room than in the back of the truck. (C) is not going to do any harm, but is not really indicated at this time. (D) is not true, as uncomplicated births are a BLS-level skill nationwide.

36. A

The correct answer this time is to respond emergently to the nearest hospital that has maternity capabilities. This is a breech delivery that places the baby at great risk for asphyxia and the mother at risk for delivery complications. The baby has to either be repositioned for a normal vaginal delivery, which is beyond the scope of EMS training, or be delivered by Caesarean section, which is a hospital procedure. You will also want to support the mother with high-flow oxygen, continue to monitor the delivery, and possibly provide airway support to the baby by inserting your hand into the birth canal.

37. B

This patient's violent outburst has no apparent cause and he must be medically evaluated. EMS will always assist police, providing it can be done safely and with a minimum amount of risk to the EMTs. Remember that the police carry weapons and are trained in dealing with violent subjects, whereas EMS is not. (C) is incorrect, since it could be considered abandonment of a seriously ill patient, and (D) is incorrect, since by removing his handcuffs he now becomes a danger to the EMTs as well as any other bystanders.

38. B

The patient should be placed in a supine position on a backboard with limbs secured with leather or vinyl cuffs. This position gives the EMT the best position to continually evaluate the patient and treat any problems as they occur. (A) is incorrect, since this patient is at an increased risk for restraint asphyxia. (C) is incorrect because the handcuffs will be forced into the small of his back; also, you will be unable to see the patient or intervene if serious conditions develop. (D) is incorrect because the patient may easily withdraw his limbs and then assault the EMTs.

39. C

The patient's behavior is abnormal and should be considered risky. After you have requested police to respond, you may then take her gently by the arm and escort her to a place where you can evaluate her more thoroughly. (A) is incorrect because her behavior is not violent at this time and she has not demonstrated a clear threat to you, bystanders, or herself. (B) is incorrect because you have not done a thorough examination to determine hypoglycemia. Just because she has had this condition in the past does not mean that this is the case at this time.

40. D

In some jurisdictions, it may be permissible to restrain without medical control. Still, to prevent a future charge of assault, battery, or false imprisonment, it is more prudent to seek medical control. The need to restrain is demonstrated by the patient's attempts to escape from the stretcher; her answers to questions indicate that she is somehow impaired. This patient must be transported to a medical facility for evaluation. Once permission from medical control is obtained, she should be restrained with the least amount of force and restraint necessary. Consequently, her wrists could be restrained to the sides of the stretcher, since she is not kicking or punching violently. Handcuffs should not routinely be used by EMS. (C) should be never be done because of the risk of asphyxiation to the patient.

CHAPTER 7

Trauma Emergencies

Topics Discussed

- The Science of Trauma and Kinetics
- The Golden Hour and Patient Prioritization
- Trauma Center Levels
- Common Traumatic Injuries
- Bleeding and Shock
- Soft Tissue Injuries and Burns
- Musculoskeletal Care
- Injuries to the Head/Spine, Eyes/Face/Neck, and Chest/Abdomen/Genitalia

The Science of Trauma

Before you arrive on the scene of a 911 call, it is important to understand the mechanisms of how injuries work. The rapid assessment of any serious injury is critical to success in patient management.

The assessment of a serious injury starts with an understanding of kinematics and velocity.

Kinematics

Kinematics refers to looking at a trauma scene and attempting to determine what injuries might have resulted from the incident that took place. Certain injury patterns occur with certain mechanisms of injury (MOI), such as:

- Whiplash of a driver, as a result of a rear- or front-end motor vehicle accident
- Abdominal injury, fractured extremities, or head injury of a pedestrian, as a result of being struck by a vehicle while walking
- Spinal injury to cervical or lumbar sections of a diver, as a result of diving headfirst into a shallow swimming pool

Similarly, low energy weapons such as knives have a different injury severity than a high energy weapon such as a gun.

Kinetic energy is the energy of a moving object. **Kinematics** is the evaluation of the accident scene to identify potential injuries that may have occurred as a result of the moving forces.

You must also look at the actual force or impact sustained by the body and soft tissues, so ask yourself the following questions:

- Was it a **soft or hard object** that struck the body?
- At what **velocity (speed)** did the object strike the person?
- Was it **one object or multiple objects** that struck the person?
- What is the **person's weight or body mass versus the weight or mass of the object struck?**

Having an understanding of how these scientific principals are at play can help predict injury patterns. In the field, this will help you determine the most appropriate facility for the given patient, i.e., level 1 versus level 3 trauma center.

Prioritization of Patients

With trauma emergencies, the goal is to get the patient to the trauma surgery center within **60 minutes of the injury**, i.e., the "**golden hour.**" Research has shown that serious trauma patients have a much higher survival rate when surgical intervention is started within that time frame.

Thus, the EMT must calculate the amount of time for the following:

- Time between the patient's injury and EMS notification
- Time spent in responding
- Time on scene assessing and treating immediate injuries
- Time required to transport the patient to the trauma center

Taking all of those factors into consideration, the EMT should determine a treatment plan, extrication process (if needed), immobilization technique, and appropriate facility for transport.

Trauma Center Levels

Determining what level of trauma center depends on not only the severity of the injury, but also what capabilities the hospital has and also if it is an adult or pediatric specialization. In general, there are four levels of trauma centers and the EMT must be familiar with what hospitals are located in their coverage area.

As an EMT, it is your job to identify the patient's level of trauma and transport to an appropriate nearby facility. In mass-casualty incidents, such as bombings, it is also important not to overwhelm one particular hospital.

Table 7.1 *Trauma Levels*

Trauma Level	Capabilities
Level 1 (highest level of trauma care certification)	• **Can provide total care, from prevention through rehabilitation** • 24-hour in-house coverage by general surgeons • Prompt availability of specialties such as orthopedic surgery, neurosurgery, anesthesiology, emergency medicine, radiology, internal medicine, plastic surgery, oral and maxillofacial, pediatric, and critical care
Level 2	• **Can initiate definitive care for all injured patients** • 24-hour immediate coverage by general surgeons, but not necessarily in-house • Specialties include orthopedic surgery, neurosurgery, anesthesiology, emergency medicine, radiology, and critical care • Cardiac surgery and hemodialysis may be referred out to a level 1 facility
Level 3	• **Can provide prompt assessment and stabilization of patients but will refer out to higher level of care hospitals** • 24-hour immediate coverage by emergency medicine physicians • Prompt availability of general surgeons and anesthesiologists (but not necessarily in-house) • Provides backup care for rural and community hospitals
Level 4	• **Can provide advanced trauma life support (ATLS) prior to transfer of patients to a higher-level trauma center** • Basic emergency department facilities and 24-hour laboratory coverage • Trauma nurse(s) and physicians available upon patient arrival • May provide surgery and critical-care services if available

Adapted from amtrauma.org

Common Types of Trauma

The most common type of trauma seen by EMS is the motor vehicle accident (MVA), also called motor vehicle collision (MVC). Falls are the second most common trauma dispatch.

Motor Vehicle Accident

There are multiple forces at work that occur when an MVA happens. Knowing the patterns will help you interpret injuries that might not be visible with the naked eye. It will also help clarify why a particular injury may be presenting with certain symptoms.

Speed matters. If a moving vehicle strikes an immovable object such as a tree (versus a moving car), the vehicle decelerates from its forward speed to zero, while the driver and passengers continue moving forward at the original rate of speed, striking the interior parts of the vehicle.

In an MVA, there are 3 strikes that occur: **car versus the object, patient versus the car,** and **organ versus the patient.** Therefore, you must have a high index of suspicion that internal injuries will be present, even if you don't see anything externally at first.

If a driver is not restrained by a seat belt and the vehicle is moving at 50 miles per hour, he will strike the steering wheel with the chest, abdomen, and pelvis. His head may continue upward into the windshield, which is constructed of double-thickness glass lined with a plastic sheet. Depending on how the vehicle is struck, the driver could have injuries in all planes of movement: lateral, rotational, anterior, and posterior.

- Approach from the front of vehicle if possible, to avoid cervical rotation.
- Communicate with the patient and ask him or her to hold as still as possible, and not turn the head.
- Inform the patient ahead of time if your partner will be taking c-spine precautions from behind the head so the patient does not inadvertently rotate the head to see what is happening.

Injury patterns can be predicted or anticipated depending on how the vehicle was struck.

There are five types of collision: frontal, broadside (T-bone), rear-end, rotational, and rollover.

A **frontal** collision between two moving vehicles is referred to as a **head-on collision**, and the force of impact is the total of both speeds. Suppose there is a head-on crash of two vehicles each doing 30 miles per hour. That is the equivalent of a single vehicle striking a tree or wall at 60 miles per hour. Watch for injuries such as "down and under" or "up and over."

- **Down-and-under**: occupant continues to move downward into the seat toward the dashboard and steering column.
  - The chest and lower extremities are often the first point of contact after striking the steering wheel or gas/brake pedals.
  - Look for lower extremities injuries such as the knee striking the dashboard, dislocated knees and hips, and fractures to the femur and/or tibia.
- **Up-and-over**: occupant continues in a forward motion, which then carries the body up and over the steering wheel.
  - The head is often the first point of contact, colliding with the windshield.
  - Look for "starring" or "bulls-eye" patterns in the glass, which would suggest that there are cranial and spinal injuries from impact.

A **broadside** (or **T-bone**) crash is a crash in which a vehicle either strikes an object sideways or is struck by another vehicle from the side. In this type of collision, there is usually more than one patient on scene, so you may need to call for additional units.

Depending on whether there is "intrusion" into the vehicle, i.e., a door is pushed inward and unable to be opened, extended extrication efforts may need to be done by the properly trained personnel.

Common injuries seen in broadside crashes include:

- **Head/neck injury**, such as whiplash from hyperextension or head strike to the window/door/other occupant
- **Chest injury**
  - Rapid compression of the thoracic wall and resulting fractured ribs, on the side that was hit in collision
  - Pulmonary contusion
  - Aorta injuries, e.g., dissection, which is life-threatening
  - Compressed and/or fractured clavicles
  - Compression fracture due to sudden tightening of the seat belt against chest wall
- **Abdominal/pelvic injury**: internal organs may have been lacerated or burst. Intrusion can compress and fracture the pelvis and dislocate the femur.
- **Entrapped limbs**: this may cause compression and crush injuries.

A **rollover** accident can be visually distracting but doesn't always cause major injuries, which can be surprising for the EMS provider. Sometimes, the occupants will self-extricate or even be ejected from the vehicle from the sheer velocity of the spinning vehicle. Those accidents which do require careful extraction by emergency personnel can cause injuries of all kinds and in all planes. Never attempt to move a patient from an unstable vehicle and be aware of scene safety at all times.

- **Shearing injury**, possible in the form of internal organs moving and tearing at their points of attachment, i.e., the aorta or liver
- **Fracture(s)**, possible from any angle, depending on what patient strikes while inside the vehicle
- **Crush injury** (vehicle comes to rest and "crushes" the patient at any point on the body); especially serious if patient was ejected as the vehicle rolled over and was crushed by the weight of the car

A **rotational** accident is when one corner of a vehicle strikes another vehicle or object, for example, when a car clips another car but they don't fully crash. The corner of the vehicle striking the object will come to a standstill while the rest of the vehicle will spin until the momentum dissipates and it finally comes to a full stop. This means that the patient inside will continue to move around and may have injuries seen in both frontal and lateral impact collisions.

A **rear-end** accident is when a vehicle strikes another vehicle from behind. This can be done at either slow or fast speeds and can involve more than two vehicles in a chain reaction. Remember that the faster a car is traveling, the more force will be exerted on all passengers, no matter which vehicle is theirs, so be prepared for multiple patients. Take spinal precautions as indicated.

Common injuries include:

- **Head/neck**: whiplash is a common complaint from one or both drivers or occupants due to rapid back and forth movement of the cervical spine. They may also have facial or head injuries from striking the windshield or headrest of the seat.
- **Chest/back**: strikes to the steering wheel, seat belt restraints locking in, and airbag deployment injuries
- **Extremities**: watch for direct and indirect forces acting up the upper and lower extremities. For example, if someone slammed on the brakes they may have ankle or leg fractures, while if they reached out with outstretched arms to prevent from going forward they may have arm fractures or dislocations.

Airbag deployment in any type of accident should be noted, i.e., whether the airbag(s) have in fact deployed and precisely which ones. Patients may complain of facial pain from the force of the airbag deployment, respiratory problems from the sudden force to the chest, or breathing problems from the inhalation of chemicals used to inflate the airbag.

If a patient self-extricates from an MVA and is found walking around prior to EMS arrival, that does not always mean he or she is fine. Adrenaline and shock have a way of masking injuries that are very serious. Therefore, it is imperative that anyone involved in an MVA have a physical and neurological exam—not only from a patient care perspective but also from a legal one.

Falls and Penetration Injury

Again, the EMT must understand how the fall occurred in order to perform a correct assessment. For example, a person who jumps from a second-floor window and lands on their feet will be at risk for serious leg and spinal injuries, while a person who falls from the same window and lands face forward will be more at risk for internal organ damage.

If full spinal immobilization is indicated, then do so. However, some falls only result in localized injuries and do not require a full spine board. Different types of splinting are reviewed later on in the chapter.

Penetration injuries from sharp objects and firearms are a specialty all their own. Fortunately, our skin is designed with multiple layers for protection of underlying organs and structures. However, depending on the size, force, and material, the skin can only protect from so much. Treatment of penetrating injuries varies depending on the object that has caused the issue, but in general, the following guidelines should be observed:

- If the object is blocking the airway, remove it carefully and manage any bleeding or suction needed and ventilate if necessary.
- If the object is still inside the skin, do not remove it as it could be acting as a type of internal tourniquet and the bleeding may be uncontrollable once removed in the field.

- Stabilize the object with gauze and bulky dressings and secure it firmly. Make sure to assess and reassess for pulse, motor, and sensation function.
- Attempt to control any bleeding that is found.

Penetrating injuries can be very distracting, but what matters most is what lies beneath and how the patient is presenting. Be prepared to manage shock symptoms and airway issues if they arise, and transport rapidly if needed.

Bleeding and Shock

External Bleeding

The average adult human has approximately 5–6 liters of blood in circulation. If blood is lost as a result of a traumatic injury, the result may be a condition called **hypoperfusion syndrome**, or traumatic shock. This condition is defined as the inadequate circulation of blood through an organ.

The sudden loss of 1 liter of blood from an average adult is considered significant, as it affects the circulatory system's ability to perfuse the organs. If blood loss continues, this can lead to devastating results. If a person has less than 2.5 liters of blood circulating, this is almost certain death, if they are not dead already.

- **Gross hemorrhage** identifies blood that can be seen to the naked eye and its growing volume. For example, if an uncontrolled femoral artery bleed is not stopped, the person will exsanguinate (bleed out) and most likely die due to the amount of blood volume lost.
- **Occult hemorrhage** is blood that cannot be seen to the naked eye. It is usually confirmed with lab tests done upon arrival at the hospital, i.e., not done in the prehospital field.

There are three types of external bleeding: arterial, venous, and capillary.

- **Arterial bleeding** occurs when an artery is lacerated and the blood spurts from the wound. This blood will be bright red as it is oxygen-rich. Arterial bleeding is more difficult to control as it is at a higher pressure.
- **Venous bleeding**, which is darker purplish in color opposite to arterial bright red because it is oxygen-poor, will flow normally or even slowly ooze rather than spurt from a wound.
- **Capillary bleeding** is usually minor and dark red in color and will often clot on its own without outside intervention.

Before the EMT considers the medical care of external bleeding, you must be sure to be wearing the proper protective equipment to assure your own safety. Depending on the amount of blood involved, that means some or all of the following: disposable gloves, masks, eye protection, and gowns.

Emergency Care of External Bleeding

A patient with a severe amount of bleeding may demand that the EMT immediately stop the loss of blood, but the airway must be secured first.

Remember, a patient without an airway will arrive at the emergency department dead. Address the airway first.

Table 7.2 *Types of Bleed*

Type of Bleed	Steps to Take
Open Venous Wound (not head or nose)	**Goal is to constrict the blood flow from the ruptured vessels and promote clotting** 1. Take a sterile dressing and apply direct pressure to the wound using a gloved hand 2. If patient is awake and able to follow commands, you can ask them to hold direct pressure 3. Elevate wound above the head and torso to help slow the flow of blood and control the bleeding 4. Add additional gauze on top of gauze as needed to stop bleeding, but be prepared to take more aggressive measures 5. Splinting using an air pressure/vacuum splint or traction splint may also help to control bleeding caused by broken bones by applying consistent pressure * If direct pressure or splinting fails to work, pressure to an extremity artery between the heart and the wound may facilitate clotting. Pressure points are located where the brachial artery crosses the humerus; radial artery crosses the wrist; and femoral artery crosses the femur.
Epistaxis ("bloody nose")	1. Have patient sit up and lean forward (leaning backward can cause aspiration) 2. Apply pressure at the bridge of the nose 3. Be prepared if blood has trickled down the back of patient's throat (may feel urge to cough or vomit); proper eye protection may lessen the risk to the provider
Ear and Nose (not spontaneous epistaxis)	**May be the result of trauma to the skull and should not be controlled by direct pressure** 1. Check for indications of underlying skull fractures: spongy feeling when palpating, obvious bone shards, "Battle sign" of bruising behind the ears, or deformities 2. Check for CSF (cerebrospinal fluid) leakage or blood leaking from ears; cover with gauze and tape to "catch" the fluid 3. Assess and calculate a GCS score—reassess every 5–10 minutes depending on severity of patient
Capillary Bleeding	**Typically very easy to control and may already have stopped bleeding prior to EMS arrival** 1. Identify all areas of bleeding and exposed wounds to make sure there is not a deeper bleed occurring 2. If wound has not already begun to clot, provide direct pressure on wound until bleeding stops 3. Place and secure bandage if necessary

Tourniquet Usage

A **tourniquet** is the most efficient way to control arterial bleeding in an extremity. A tourniquet is a bandage at least 4 inches wide placed between the heart and approximately 2 inches above the wound. When applied and tightened, it will stop all blood flow to the wound distal to the device.

- Consequences may include nerve and tissue damage secondary to the stoppage of oxygenated blood flow to the tissues and cells beyond the application point.
- If done correctly, can be in place for up to 2 hours without causing irreversible tissue or nerve damage.
- Receiving facility should be advised immediately that the tourniquet has been applied and "TQ" should be written on the patient's forehead or other visible location, especially in a mass casualty situation.

Tourniquets have become required equipment on both BLS and ALS units nationwide. While most services utilize commercial tourniquets such as CAT, Sof-T, Israeli bandages, or SWAT-T, it is also possible to improvise and make tourniquets if necessary.

To make a tourniquet:

- Use a wide bandage (never rope or wire that could cut into the tissue and cause necrosis)
- Tie the bandage with a half hitch and place a stick or bandage scissors on top of the knot, then complete the knot by tying an opposite half hitch to complete a square knot
- Twist the stick or scissors to tighten the bandage until the bleeding stops and then secure the stick or scissors with another bandage
- A quick tourniquet that can be improvised is the use of the blood pressure cuff (monitor for air loss)

Regardless of whether it is a commercial or improvised unit, there are a few rules when using a tourniquet:

- Never loosen it once applied, since doing so could result in severe shock (blood rushes from the brain to fill the injured extremity).
- Never apply it directly over a joint.
- Know the specific features of your service's equipment beforehand so that you don't need to "read the directions" in a true emergency.

Hemostatic Agents

Hemostatic agents are substances used to control injured blood vessels, which are typically arterial because of their hard-to-control nature when lacerated. These agents work by contracting tissue to seal the injured blood vessels (anti-hemorrhagic).

Originally used mainly in the military, studies have shown there is a usage in the prehospital field as well. There are commercial brands that come in different formats to help EMS professionals, such as:

- Impregnated gauze
- Free flowing powder
- Granule packets

Not all units nationwide will carry this, so it is up to the EMT to be properly trained in its usage if present on their truck.

Internal Bleeding

Internal bleeding is more problematic for the EMT since it is not always apparent, yet may lead to severe hypovolemic shock and death. This is especially true when internal organs in the torso have been ruptured due to severe trauma such as an automobile accident or fall. Blunt force trauma can also be caused by blast injuries.

Suspicion of serious internal bleeding may be deduced from the mechanism of injury and signs and symptoms that the EMT finds when performing the trauma assessment. These signs and symptoms would include:

- Pain, tenderness, swelling, or discoloration of the suspected site
- Bleeding from the mouth, rectum, vagina, or other body orifices
- Blood in vomit, urine, or stool
- Tenderness, rigidity, and distension of the abdomen

Treatment of internal bleeding treats the hypoperfusion syndrome that results. Suspicion of internal bleeding will raise the priority of the transport, and the "golden hour" becomes much more critical in these types of cases. Transport to the proper facility rapidly, ideally one with surgical capabilities.

Emergency Care of Shock

As the body's own mechanisms respond to attempt to heal and compensate for a traumatic injury, these systems may be overwhelmed. Serious harm may occur as a result.

Hemorrhagic shock occurs when the volume of blood becomes insufficient to provide oxygen and nutrients to the cells or remove waste products from the cells. This condition may lead to serious organ damage or death.

The EMT must also be aware of the signs and symptoms of hypovolemic shock, which include:

- Anxiety or altered mental status
- General weakness or dizziness
- Tachypnea and tachycardia
- Cool, pale, and clammy skin
- Delayed capillary refill (longer than 2 seconds)
- Nausea and vomiting
- Dilated pupils that are sluggish in response to light

The classic sign of hypovolemic shock is dropping blood pressure. This is considered a late sign, so treatment measures should be in place before it develops. With children, since they have a lower blood volume than adults, a dropping blood pressure may indicate that they are close to death, and aggressive treatment is necessary.

Treatment for hypoperfusion syndrome includes the following:

- Maintain the airway, ventilating if necessary
- Administer high-flow oxygen
- Control external bleeding
- Elevate the lower extremities 8–12 inches
- Splint any suspected fractures
- Prevent heat loss by covering the patient with blankets
- Expedite transport to a trauma center if indicated

If your protocols allow, and with the approval of medical control, consider application of a pneumatic antishock garment called a PASG (*but very few agencies still use these devices*).

Soft Tissue Injuries and Burns

Soft Tissue Injuries

Soft tissue injuries are injuries to skin, muscle, tendons, and/or ligaments. In other words, these are not direct fractures to bone or injuries to internal organs. However, soft tissue injuries are not always isolated, i.e., they may occur alongside bone fractures or internal underlying damage.

Recall that the skin has three layers: the outermost **epidermis**; the **dermis**, which contains the oil glands and hair follicles; and the **subcutaneous layer**, which contains fatty deposits and helps to provide cushioning and/or temporary protection.

The degree of soft tissue injury is directly related to the number of skin layers involved. For example:

- If we are referring to a burn, we need to know which layers of skin have been affected to determine the depth and severity.

- If we are referring to a laceration or avulsion, we want to know the depth or layer of skin that has been injured. There may be a superficial abrasion within the top layer of the skin, while an avulsion may go all the way down to the subcutaneous layer.

Treatment protocols will necessitate that the EMT can recognize these as well.

Closed Injuries

A closed injury is when the epidermis remains intact and there is no external bleeding. There are three types of closed injury.

- In a **contusion**, the cells and smaller blood vessels are damaged below the epidermis from some type of trauma, and blood pools in the tissues causing a purplish discoloration. This area is often swollen and painful to the touch.

- A **hematoma** involves laceration of a larger blood vessel, either an artery or a vein, and results in a large pool of blood beneath the epidermal layer.

- A **crushing injury** is a closed tissue injury that may cause internal organ rupture; the accompanying bleeding may be so severe as to cause hypoperfusion syndrome (shock).

Emergency medical care for these types of injuries involves appropriate body substance isolation, airway and ventilatory support, treatment for shock, and rapid transport. If the injury involves an extremity, it is often helpful for both treatment of hypovolemia and pain management to splint the extremity. Since these types of injuries cannot be well managed in the prehospital setting, rapid transport to a trauma center is always indicated (remember the "golden hour").

Open Injuries

Open injuries are open wounds with external bleeding.

Table 7.3 *Soft Tissue Wounds*

Open Wound Type	Characteristics
Abrasion	• **Epidermal layer damaged by shearing or scraping** • Very painful, though superficial injury • Causes minimal blood loss • Because of larger area involved, more prone to infection than smaller area wounds
Laceration	• **Break in the skin, of varying depth** • *Linear* laceration is an incision caused by a sharp object, while *irregular* laceration is caused by blunt trauma • Depending on depth and location, bleeding may be minor to severe • The deeper the wound, the greater the danger of infection, as bacteria may have been introduced deep into the tissues by the object causing the laceration • Consider use of hemostatic agent if indicated
Avulsion	• **Flap of skin or tissue torn off by a traumatic force** • Very painful • Causes significant blood loss • Fold back flap of skin into original position if possible
Amputation	• **Complete separation of a distal extremity or part from the extremity or trunk** • May cause minimal bleeding if it is clean cut (rather than a tearing off) • Attempt to find amputated item to transport to hospital with patient
Penetration/Puncture	• **Deep intrusion into soft tissue by any object, e.g., a bullet or knife** • May cause minimal or no external bleeding, but depth of the injury may produce significant internal bleeding • If object is still protruding from body, stabilize it with gauze and secure it with tape so it doesn't move around during transport and cause further damage • Search and identify all wounds (don't forget the back and sides)
Open Crush	• **Crushed body part due to pressure from a heavy object** • May be open or closed • Greater danger is to the underlying organs and tissues • Call for additional personnel to remove crushing object if present; also consider ALS • Depending on location and time of crush, be prepared for traumatic cardiac arrest

Management of soft tissue injuries is as follows:

- Your first concern is to protect yourself from the dangers of bloodborne pathogens. A massive trauma scenario involving large volumes of blood loss requires more extensive precautions than a simple finger laceration. Precautions may include:
  - Full body gown, mask
  - Eye protection, gloves
  - Shoe coverings

- Once the scene is safe and precautions have been taken, you must secure the patient's airway and provide ventilatory support. In the presence of a gross traumatic injury, some EMTs will focus on the injury site and neglect to check an airway (called a *distracting injury*). It is human nature to want to address all injuries at once, but remember that a patient without an airway will arrive at the ER dead.

- Once the airway and breathing are secure, the area of bleeding must be exposed and the rest of the body thoroughly checked for other wounds, including exit wounds.
  - For legal reasons, if the wounds are caused by bullets, be careful *not* to document each wound as such in your PCR, i.e., note only that you found "multiple wounds" and describe location and severity of each.
  - In calls where weapons were involved, police may be involved to secure the scene. There may also be a potential criminal case where you may be called to testify.
  - To clarify even further, EMTs are not trained to be ballistic experts, nor are they trained as coroners, so they do not have the expertise to properly identify which wound is which—lawyers will point this out if the case goes to court.

- Finally, with an open wound, prevention of further bacterial contamination becomes a concern. Sterilize things as much as possible to minimize the danger of further contamination by doing the following:
  - Open packages only as items are needed.
  - Use rubbing alcohol (at least 60% strength) to clean off the equipment prior to usage.

- Once bleeding has been controlled, dress open wounds with dry sterile dressings and secure with clean bandaging materials such as muslin cravats or self-securing bandaging material.
  - Remember that blood loss leads to shock and that the treatment of hypovolemic syndrome must always be a concern.
  - Refer back to the previous section on bleeding and shock management for review.

Following treatment of a severe trauma patient, it is always prudent to remain out of service until the unit has been properly decontaminated. Providers may choose at their discretion (and with approval from supervisors or dispatch) to return to the station for a shower and clothing change. Any clothing that has been exposed to blood must be considered contaminated and washed properly, in accordance with local guidelines for dealing with bodily fluid–contaminated objects.

There is no set amount of time that is "required" to be out of service when decontaminating your truck unit. Depending on what's required, it could be as little as just wiping down any visible blood from the windows/seats/equipment or as much as fully disinfecting and mopping the truck. You could be out of service from 10 minutes to over an hour.

Whatever amount of cleaning that needs to be done, it must first be cleared with your supervisor or dispatch center. The expectation is that your unit should be back in service within a reasonable amount of time and ready to take additional emergency calls as soon as possible.

Special Situations and Treatments

Some wounds, due to their location on the body, present special situations and require special treatments.

- **Chest wound** accompanied by a gurgling sound and frothy blood indicates that the lung has been penetrated.
  - Could lead to a severely collapsed lung or pneumothorax (known as *sucking chest wounds*).
  - If collapse is so severe as to cause the organs in the chest to shift position, e.g., tracheal deviation (called a *tension pneumothorax*), that is a life-threatening situation requiring rapid treatment and transport.
  - Treatment is dressing with an occlusive dressing, which will block airflow into the collapsed pleural space; always administer oxygen, as the patient will almost always have compromised breathing.
- **Abdominal injury** accompanied by protruding organs (called an *evisceration injury*) is always serious. Do not touch the organs or attempt to put them back inside the abdomen. Treatment is coverage of the wound with a sterile dressing, thoroughly moistened with sterile water or saline. Transport immediately.
- **Impaled object** in the body should not be removed, as it typically tourniquets the blood internally (exceptions include an object through the cheek, an object that would interfere with chest compressions, or an object that would interfere with transport). Treatment is contacting medical control for advice on how to proceed, but oftentimes that includes securing the object, controlling any peripheral bleeding, and transporting.
- **Extremity amputation** is treated as any other open wound.
  - May be partial or complete
  - May produce tremendous blood loss, depending on location
  - Has a psychological component for the EMT
  - Treatment is immediate transport to the emergency department; if possible, locate and transport the amputated part as well, for possible reattachment.
    - Wrap amputated part in a sterile dressing and place in a plastic bag.
    - Place plastic bag on an ice pack, to keep cool; **do not place amputated part directly on ice as it will freeze.**

    − If amputation is partial, stabilize as best as possible; **do not attempt to complete amputation**.

- **Neck injury** poses unique challenges in both securing a bandage and also making sure the airway stays patent. If there is frothy bleeding, this may indicate injury to both the airway and blood vessels in the neck. Treatment is an occlusive dressing, which will prevent an embolism from entering the circulatory system and causing cardiac/respiratory arrest.

An **occlusive dressing** is by definition a sterile dressing of non-breathing material that covers a wound on all sides. In some injuries (e.g., a sucking chest wound) the occlusive dressing is modified by taping only 3 sides so that excess air in the thoracic cavity is able to escape on the fourth side ("burping").

There are commercial premade options, but there are a variety of materials you can use to make your own:

- **Not gauze** (too breathable, i.e., air can permeate)!
- Paper or plastic packaging from a gauze pad (with gauze discarded)
- Plastic food wrap

Whatever material is used, place it directly over the wound, tape on 3 sides, and leave the fourth side open for the excess air in the thoracic cavity to escape ("burping").

Burns

Burn Depth

Burns are classified according to the depth of the injured tissue. Even though the current literature lists the three categories as superficial, partial thickness, and full thickness, EMT and hospital staff may still refer to these as first, second, and third degree.

- A **first-degree** (superficial) burn involves only the epidermis.
  - Characterized by a reddening of the skin and local pain
  - Example: ordinary sunburn
- A **second-degree** (partial-thickness) burn involves both the epidermis and dermis, but not the underlying tissue.
  - Accompanied by intense pain and blistering of the skin
  - Skin may be bright red to white
  - Example: sunburn that has fluid-filled blisters

- A **third-degree** (full-thickness) burn involves all three layers of skin and possibly underlying muscles, bones, tissues, and organs.

  – Characterized by charred, dry, and leathery skin

  – May cause little or no pain where skin is burned if sensory nerves were damaged or destroyed

  – Peripheral areas usually have lesser degree burns with extreme pain

Rule of Nines

The overall survivability of a burn patient is contingent not only upon the depth/type of burn, but also on the amount of skin surface (body surface area [BSA]) involved.

The **rule of nines** was developed to assist EMS in relaying to the receiving facility how much BSA is involved in the burn injury. There are 11 body areas, each of which contains approximately 9% of the body's overall area. For an adult, they are broken down as follows:

Body Part	% of Body Surface Area
Head and neck	9
Chest	9
Abdomen	9
Front of each leg (two areas)	18
Back of each leg (two areas)	18
Arms (two areas)	18
Upper back	9
Lower back	9

*Note: These BSAs add up to 99%; the genitalia comprise the remaining 1%.

Suppose a patient sustains burns on his face and both arms. Each arm is 9%, for a total of 18%. The front of the face is 4.5% (half of 9%). Thus, the total BSA is 22.5%.

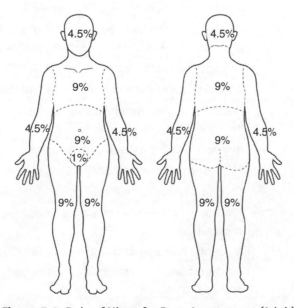

Figure 7.1 *Rule of Nines for Burn Assessment (Adult)*

The pediatric rule of nines will be discussed in chapter 8.

An alternative method for measuring burns is the **palmar** method. The patient's palm and fingers equal approximately 1% of BSA burned. It is not to be used on large surface area burns, however, where the rule of nines would be more appropriate.

TEST YOURSELF 7.1

What percentage is this patient burned?

A 45-year-old female has sustained some burns after a cooking accident where hot oil splashed up from the pan onto her. She has sustained burns to her hands, anterior forearms, and upper chest. What percentage of her body has been burned?

Burn Severity

Burn severity is also gauged by location. Once the type of burn and the BSA affected have been determined, the EMT can determine the severity of the injury.

Burns to the face and torso are highly challenging given the patient's risk of inhaling any products of combustion, leading to possible swelling of the airway and fluid buildup in the lungs.

Table 7.4 *Severity of Burns*

Minor Burn	Superficial burn covering <50% of BSA
	Second-degree burn covering <15% of BSA
	Third-degree burn covering <2% of BSA
Moderate Burn	Any third-degree burn involving 2–10% of BSA, unless it involves the hands, feet, face, genitalia, or upper chest
	Any second-degree burn involving 15–30% of BSA
	Any first-degree burn involving >50% of BSA
Severe Burn	Any third-degree burn involving the hands, feet, face, or genitalia
	Any burn involving respiratory damage
	Third-degree burns involving >10% of BSA
	Second-degree burns involving >30% of BSA
	Any burns complicated by painful, swollen, or deformed extremities
	Moderate burns to pediatric and geriatric patients
	Any burns which encompass an entire body part, such as an arm, leg, chest, etc.

Suppose a male patient has a sunburn that covers all of his body except the area covered by a bathing suit. EMS would identify him as having a superficial burn covering 70–80% of his BSA. That is considered a moderate burn injury, not a minor burn.

Treatment

Treatment of burns will range from minor wound management using sterile gauze to emergent transport to a certified burn center. Severity depends on the type, size, location, and depth of the burn. However, there are some universal steps to take no matter the type of burn inflicted.

First, stop the burning process.

- Remove any burnt clothing and all jewelry.
- Pour copious amounts of water or saline onto the burnt area.
- Be alert for airway compromise if there has been exposure to any products of combustion.

Second, use extreme caution to prevent any infection.

- Create as sterile an environment for the patient as possible.
- Once cooled, cover burnt areas with loose dressings.
- Do not ever break blisters.
- Do not ever apply ointment, lotion, or antiseptics in the emergency care setting.

Third, address the patient's temperature, since severe burn can affect the body's ability to regulate core temperature.

- Manage any hypothermia or dehydration.
- Give supplemental oxygen therapy as needed.

Chemical and electrical burns have additional considerations:

- Treat **chemical burns** by flushing with water or with fluids recommended for that particular chemical (try to read label or manufacturer's safety data sheet [MSDS]).
  - Brush any caustic powder off the skin before flushing.
  - Take care not to allow the runoff fluid from washing to injure unaffected body parts.
  - Never attempt to neutralize a chemical burn using another chemical, such as applying a base to an acid burn. The resulting chemical reaction can create heat that will further burn the patient.
  - You may also ask if the patient knows the chemical name—if yes, then it may be looked up in the Emergency Response Guidebook (ERG). This book allows the provider to not only look up the chemical's properties, but also to see first-aid responses and how far away a provider should be if there is a leak or spill.

- **Electrical burns** are a concern for the safety of the responding crew.
  - Be sure that the person is not still energized by contact with the electrical object that caused the injury; if you are unsure, do not touch the patient (for your own safety).
  - Once you have determined that the patient is safe to touch, treat the wound as you would any burn.
  - Contact with an electrical object may cause both an entrance and exit wound, as the electricity goes to ground.
  - Electrocution may cause cardiac arrhythmia, so have the AED ready to use in case the victim's heart begins to fibrillate.

Injuries to the Musculoskeletal System

Injuries to the musculoskeletal system of the body are among the most challenging to the EMT. The principles of this type of care are important to understand since trauma patients will rarely present with a textbook example of a musculoskeletal injury. The EMT will have to improvise treatment utilizing these principles.

In order to implement a treatment plan for this type of injury, a study of the **mechanism of injury** (MOI) is necessary.

Types of Force

The NREMT curriculum mentions three types of force that cause injury.

- In **direct force**, the injury occurs at the point of impact. If a window falls onto someone's forearm and fractures the radius, this is an example of a direct force injury.
- In **indirect force**, the injury occurs away from the point of impact. An example of indirect force would be when a subject falls and lands on his feet and the force of the landing causes his hip to dislocate.
- **Twisting force**, as the name implies, occurs when one part of an extremity remains stationary while another part rotates. The best example of this is a sprained ankle.

Types of Bone Injury

There are two types of bone and joint injury.

- **Open** fracture, sprain, or strain: broken bone or torn tissue that has a break in the continuity of the skin
- **Closed** fracture, sprain, or strain: broken bone or torn tissue that has no break in the skin

The signs and symptoms of a bone or joint injury are:

- Deformity
- Pain
- Grating

- Swelling
- Discoloration
- Exposed bone ends
- Locked joint

Emergency care is to splint the injury, apply cold to reduce swelling, and elevate the extremity to reduce the pain, as well as treat for shock. Because an open fracture is a "combination injury," it requires treatment of both the broken bone/damaged joint and the accompanying wound.

Splinting

Management of musculoskeletal injuries involves a science known as splinting—immobilization of a broken bone or damaged joint, as well as any adjacent joints. A properly applied splint will help to prevent further damage to tissues irritated by the broken bone ends. Splinting will also minimize the danger that a closed injury may progress to an open injury, further complicating patient care and resulting in a much longer recovery period.

Prior to applying a splint, distal pulse, motor, and sensation must be assessed in order to compare these vital signs once the splint has been applied. Compare the injured side to the non-injured side, especially with regard to length. The splint must immobilize the area where the EMT suspects the break has occurred, as well as the adjacent joints. A suspected mid-shaft tibia fracture must not only immobilize the mid-shaft area of the bone, but also the ankle joint and knee joint.

Prior to application of any splint, clothing must be removed or cut away. In the case of the lower extremities, shoes and boots must be removed to assure proper application of a splint as well as assessment of distal neural vital signs. If the fracture is open, the wounds must be dressed with a sterile dressing prior to splint application. If the extremity is severely deformed or if the distal area is cyanotic and pulses and sensation are absent, then the limb must be realigned with gentle traction prior to splinting. After splinting any injury, always make sure to go back and reassess distal pulse, motor, and sensation.

Types of Splints

There are many types of splints, including improvised splints used in wilderness EMS. Basically, a splint is any object that immobilizes the suspected injury and adjacent joints.

The splints most common to EMS are the *rigid board splints*, which come in a variety of sizes. These boards are then secured in whatever configuration is necessary with the use of cravats or straps. Variations of these include the vinyl splints with rigid spines that secure quickly with Velcro™.

Other examples are:

- A **long spine board** can immobilize the entire body.
- A **vacuum or air pressure splint** can provide pressure uniformly to the extremity (useful in wound management as well).

- **Traction splints** provide continuous traction of the lower extremities and are often indicated by protocol for management of closed femur fractures. A traction splint helps to alleviate pain by preventing the broken bone ends from aggravating the surrounding tissue.

- **SAM splints** are pieces of aluminum strips that are enclosed in a flexible foam padding. This makes them easily moldable to various shapes to accommodate the extremities, and they are very lightweight.

- A **PASG** (or MAST trousers) can immobilize the entire lower body including the pelvis, but it is rarely used in practice today.

Finally, many ordinary objects can be adapted for splinting, such as pillows, large towels, and large magazines. However, no matter what material used, always remember to assess and reassess PMS (pulse, motor, and sensation functions) before and after splinting has been applied. Readjust as necessary.

Injuries to the Head and Spine

With injuries to the head or spine, EMS should pay close attention to the mechanism of injury and should visualize what may have happened to the body of the patient.

- The **brain** is responsible for operating the multiple systems of the human body. It receives sensory information and sends electrical impulses to the organs, muscles, and tissues via the nervous system.

- The **spinal cord**, which runs from the base of the brain down the back, is the main transmission line for these actions. If it is damaged or severed as a result of trauma, these systems may be compromised. The spinal cord is surrounded and protected by the bony spinal column, which is composed of 33 bones called *vertebrae*.

Injury to the spinal cord may be caused by the following types of scenarios:

- **Spinal cord compression** due to significant force applied to the top of the head (as in a person diving headfirst into an empty swimming pool)

- **Spinal column and spinal cord damage** due to excessive motion (as in a sports injury)

- **Spinal column distraction** (the pulling apart of adjacent vertebrae) due to excessive stretching (as in hanging by the neck)

If you suspect spinal injury upon arrival at the scene, you will need to perform half or full immobilization utilizing a cervical collar.

As a result of new research, many EMTs are being given clearance to perform "spinal clearance" in the field. This means that if a patient does not fit certain criteria or have complaints of spinal injury, full immobilization may not be required.

Make sure that you are familiar with the local protocols of your EMS service, but gone are the days where every patient gets a backboard blindly. (In fact, it has been proven that doing so may have caused more harm than good.)

Head Injuries

Injuries to the head present a special challenge to the EMT. The scalp is extremely vascular and any open wound will cause a large amount of bleeding. Be aware that they typically look worse than they are; clean the wound with saline and examine closely.

A closed wound from blunt force trauma may cause bleeding inside the cranial compartment, causing increasing pressure inside the skull and complicating breathing and circulation. Keep in mind that in addition to trauma, some medical conditions, such as stroke, may give the same signs and symptoms as head trauma.

The EMT should suspect a brain injury when any of the following are present during the primary or focused assessment:

- Altered or decreasing mental status
- Irregular breathing
- Bleeding or bruising to the head
- Blood or fluid (cerebrospinal fluid) leaking from the ears, eyes, nose, or mouth
- Bruising around the eyes (raccoon eyes)
- Bruising behind the ears (Battle sign)
- Any neurological disability; nausea and vomiting; pupils of different sizes with altered mental status
- Seizure activity
- Feel for "spongy" areas, as this could be underlying fracture

Proper treatment of suspected skull fracture or brain injury is critical.

- Expedite transport to a trauma center immediately.
- Any head injury is assumed to involve the cervical spine, so immobilize the head and spine.
- Closely monitor the patient for abrupt changes in mental status and vital signs.
- Control any bleeding from the head as you would with any open wound, but do not apply pressure to an open or depressed skull wound since that would risk pushing a bone fragment into the brain or increasing the intercranial pressure.

Spinal Injuries

As you perform the assessment, the suspicion of a spinal cord injury rises significantly if any of the following signs or symptoms are present:

- Tenderness or pain in the back or neck
- Pain when the neck or back is moved
- Intermittent pain in the spinal column or legs independent of motion or palpation
- Any open injuries to the back or neck
- Numbness, tingling, or weakness in the extremities
- Loss of sensation or motion in the extremities
- Incontinence

If the spinal cord injury is located in the upper cervical vertebrae, then the ability to breathe or move the extremities may be compromised and you must be prepared to intervene to correct these conditions.

If a spinal injury is suspected and the patient is able to respond, it is imperative to ask if any back or neck pain is present, if the fingers and toes can be moved without pain, and if anything can be felt when you touch the extremities.

Following inspection and palpation of the neck, back, and extremities, and as part of the focused trauma assessment, ask the patient to complete two important tests to determine if there is communication from their brain to their extremities. This is achieved by asking the patient to complete the following commands and noting if there is equal strength in each extremity, if the movement causes pain, and whether or not the patient is able to complete the task.

- Ask the patient to grab your hands and squeeze very hard.
- With your hands pushing gently on the soles of the patient's feet, ask the patient to push down and then point the toes toward the head.

In case of a possible injury, the spinal cord must be immobilized in a neutral (straight) "eyes forward" position. To do this, take the head in both hands and hold it gently so that it is aligned with the spine. You can also use your first and middle fingers to perform a modified jaw thrust to secure a patent airway. This stabilization must be maintained until the patient is secured to a spine board. Once the patient is secured in this manner, has a patent airway, is breathing, has a palpable carotid pulse, and has no gross hemorrhage, then the remainder of the initial assessment can be performed.

Applying a Cervical Collar

Once the head and neck have been assessed by sight and touch, a **rigid cervical collar** (c-collar) should be applied to assist with maintaining stabilization. The c-collar must be the correct size for the patient and must be properly applied or more harm can result.

The collar must hold the head and chin up in the neutral position without hyperextending the neck. It must touch the skin on the chest and back, as well as the chin and back of the neck. To properly size a c-collar, follow the steps listed below:

1. Obtain a lateral view of the patient's head while your partner maintains the neutral in-line position.

2. With fingers outstretched, place all fingers including your thumb next to each other with no space in between.

3. Pinky finger side down, rest your outstretched hand on the base of the patient's shoulder.

4. Looking at the patient's chin, draw an imaginary straight line with your eyes.

5. Count the number of fingers it takes to meet with that imaginary straight line. For example, if your middle finger matches the line, you have three fingers worth of space to measure with on the collar.

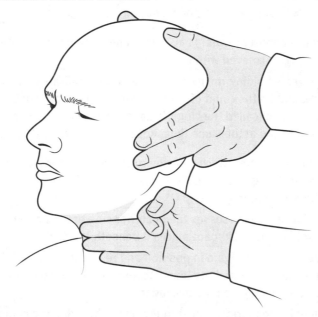

Figure 7.2 *Measuring for Cervical-Collar Height*

If you are using a c-collar that is adjustable, follow the manufacturer's guidelines to find the appropriate measurement tool on the collar itself. Place your fingers in the specified space to determine the size of the collar so it matches the number of fingers you have previously measured with. Sizes will range from "no-neck" to "tall." Secure the collar in the measured selection.

If using a nonadjustable collar, the sizing process is still the same, however you must identify which collar to use. They will be individually labeled with sizes. Because this equates to having multiple individual pieces, most systems do not utilize these, rather opting for an all-in-one adjustable collar.

Securing to a Long Backboard

When the initial assessment is complete and the c-collar has been placed, the patient is then secured to a long backboard (LBB) (or **spine board**) as follows:

Table 7.5 *Securing a Patient in Full Immobilization*

Step Number	Procedure
1	With patient laying supine, one EMT places the board next to the patient
2	One EMT continues to hold the c-spine, while the second EMT places the c-collar; if this has already been done, move on to step 3
3	Kneeling on the opposite side of where the LBB is placed, the second EMT crosses the patient's arms over the chest (as an X) so they are safely out of the way during the logroll maneuver * Ideally a third provider is also on scene to help with the next steps, but this can be achieved with two providers.
4	Whoever is holding the patient's head then confirms that everyone is ready, and on the count of 3 all providers roll the patient on their side toward them (called the "logroll maneuver"); the person holding the head rolls the head at the same time, keeping it aligned with the spine * It doesn't matter which side you roll toward, as long as everyone does the same thing in unison. If there is an injury, however, it is advisable to roll to the uninjured side.
5	One EMT quickly assesses the posterior side of the patient, and the EMT controlling the backboard places it beneath the patient
6	Once everyone is again in position and ready, the EMT holding the head again counts to 3 and the team proceeds to roll the patient to the supine position, this time on the backboard
7	Patient is then properly positioned on the board at the command of the EMT holding cervical stabilization; everyone must make coordinated movements to avoid excessive spinal movement
8	The patient is then secured to the board using a minimum of three straps, one across the chest, one across the pelvis, and one across the legs
9	The patient's head is then secured to the board using an approved device, usually head blocks and Velcro™ straps (check to see what your employer uses)
10	All distal neurological signs are checked again, and the patient, now properly splinted, is placed onto the stretcher, secured with further stretcher straps, and moved to ambulance for transport
*11	*If patient is found in a sitting position, a short spine board or intermediate transport device such as a Kendrick™ Extrication Device (KED) is used to remove them from the immediate area to a long backboard

When dealing with head or spinal injury, there are some special considerations:

- Decide whether to extricate the patient (from car, etc.) using the **time-consuming method of full spinal and head immobilization** or the more **rapid method using minimal immobilization**. The rapid method is more appropriate for unsafe situations (e.g., fire), unstable patients (e.g., not breathing), and patients who may be blocking access to a more critically injured patient.

- Decide whether to remove a sport bike or motorcycle helmet. Current protocols advise the following:

  - Remove any face guards and shields for assessment. (If at a sporting event, the team medic or coach may have a special key to deflate the pads inside.)

  - Leave the helmet on unless it is necessary to ventilate a patient or treat a severe, bleeding wound. Perform spinal stabilization with the helmet in place.

  - If removal of the helmet is necessary to prevent a potentially life-threatening condition, do it in two steps: one EMT stabilizes the head/neck, while the second EMT uses the hands to spread the helmet wide, push up, and lift off with minimal movement and strain on the head/neck.

Injuries to the Eyes, Face, and Neck

Eye Injuries

Injuries to the eye are almost always considered serious since they may have long-term consequences to the quality of life of a victim of trauma. In assessing trauma to the eyes, in addition to palpating for broken bones you should use your diagnostic penlight to determine the reactivity of the pupils to light and compare the responses from each eye to the other. Also, the patient should be able to track the light with the eyes without moving the head, and the tracking should be smooth for both eyes.

Often, foreign objects will take up residence in the eye. Small particles of dust and other foreign matter are usually removed by flushing the eyeball with sterile water or saline. Chemicals and irritants splashed into the eyes can also be removed by flushing. This can be done in a myriad of ways, including:

- Have the patient splash water into both eyes over a bowl or other receptacle such as an emesis bin

- Have the patient turn the head with the affected eye down laterally, then pour sterile water down in a stream over the eyes

- Use a nasal cannula connected to saline and placed over the bridge of the nose to irrigate both eyes:

  - Connect the NC to an IV set and a 1-liter bag of saline instead of oxygen

  - Nasal prongs rest over the medial edge of the eye socket

  - Open the IV set to flow and allow saline to come through

If there is a penetrating injury to the eye, the object is not removed, but secured in place with bandages and dressings. In this type of injury to the eye, both eyes are always covered so that the parallel motion of the uninjured eye does not cause the injured eye to move. In the case of an avulsed eyeball, do not attempt to replace the eye, but cover the eyeball with a moist sterile dressing and a clean paper cup and bandage them in place to protect the eye. Once again, cover the other eye as well.

Face Injuries

Injuries to the face are treated in the same way as other injuries, with the exception that an impaled object through the cheek may be removed by the EMT in the field in order to facilitate management of the airway. Remember that because of the extensive vasculature of the face and head, injuries to these areas will bleed profusely.

If an airway needs to be established and there is facial trauma, avoid placement of an NPA, as it could protrude into the cranial cavity.

Neck Injuries

Injuries to the neck may involve the great vessels leading to the brain, as well as injury to the airway. Bubbling and gurgling of a neck wound are indications that the injury not only involves the blood vessels, but also the airway. This type of wound requires an occlusive dressing to prevent outside air from entering the blood vessel and causing an air embolism.

If you suspect cervical spine injury an appropriately sized c-collar should be placed, but be aware that if one section of the spine is compromised then other sections may be as well.

Injuries to the Chest, Abdomen, and Genitalia

Chest Injuries

If the assessment of a trauma victim reveals paradoxical motion of the rib cage, combined with pain and crepitus of the ribs, that is an indication of a condition called **flail chest**, defined as ≥2 ribs broken in at least two places. The **paradoxical motion**, or area that falls when the chest rises and rises when chest falls, is caused by the broken or flailed area floating freely on the chest wall.

A flail chest is a major trauma, and transportation to a level 1 trauma center should be expedited. Treatment is with high-flow oxygen via non-rebreather. Be alert for respiratory failure, which will require assistance with ventilations.

Chest injury that is bubbling is called a **sucking chest wound** and, like a neck wound, must be dressed with an occlusive dressing to prevent air from entering the pleural space and increasing the likelihood of a pneumothorax. These occlusive dressings may be waterproof thin-film-type dressings or lubricated gauze pads. In an emergency, commercial plastic wrap can also be used.

Closed chest wounds are especially dangerous, especially if they involve the heart or the great vessels leading to and from the heart. A serious condition known as **cardiac tamponade**, caused by blunt trauma to the heart, occurs when the sac around the heart (pericardium) fills with blood and places pressure on the heart. Since there is no basic intervention that can be done in the field, if the EMT suspects this type of injury the patient is a load and go.

The EMT should be especially alert for trauma patients who spit or cough up blood, as these patients have a higher suspicion of a closed chest injury involving the heart or lungs.

Abdominal Injuries

In the abdominal cavity, there are multiple organs that are described as hollow or solid. Damage to either type of organ will lead to issues not only with the organ itself, but also with the surrounding tissues.

- **Hollow organs**, such as the bladder and stomach, contain acids that help digest or break down substances in the body.
  - If these organs become ruptured and discharge digestive products into the peritoneal space, patients are at increased risk of infection of the abdominal cavity.
  - For example, if the bladder is lacerated, urine is acidic to a certain extent and bacteria will be released. This acidic and bacteria mixture will then touch or coat other organs and tissues surrounding it, causing irritation.
  - Another example is the stomach, where there are acids (gastric) and broken-down food particles. If the stomach is lacerated or burst, these substances would then "float" all around the abdominal cavity and cause inflammation.
- **Solid organs**, such as the liver and spleen, are very vascular in nature, with multiple veins and arteries that populate the tissue.
  - If these organs become damaged, the result will be bleeding into the surrounding tissues. It is entirely possible for someone to exsanguinate (bleed out) into their abdominal cavity, as it is a large area that blood can collect into.
  - For example, a liver laceration can be a very serious event, as it is a large organ with multiple veins and arteries involved.

Regardless, if there is fluid collection of blood or otherwise that can be seen by the naked eye, the EMT must take note and expedite transport.

Some signs and symptoms are as follows:

- Rigidity and tenderness of the abdomen are an indication of potential fluid buildup underneath the skin.
- Leaking fluid requires immediate attention.
  - If it is a yellow color, it may be urine.
  - If it is a brown color, it may be a damaged organ responsible for holding feces, such as the intestines.
  - If it is a reddish, blood-tinged color, it may be damage to a solid organ.

- If the injury has exposed the intestines and they are protruding from the wound (called an **abdominal evisceration**), do the following:
  - Drape the intestines with moist sterile dressings.
  - Irrigate with sterile water or saline.
  - Secure the dressing on all four sides.
  - Transport immediately. Do not attempt to push the intestines back into the cavity.

Finally, keep in mind that pain can be felt in the abdomen in a variety of ways. However, some common symptoms follow:

Table 7.6 *Types of Abdominal Pain*

Pain Type	Key Facts
Visceral Pain	• Dull, achy in nature • Typically intermittent • Patient may not be able to identify where pain is coming from
Parietal Pain	• Sharp, stabbing • Typically localized in nature • Patient can often directly identify where pain is coming from
Referred Pain	• Unique, in that pain is felt "elsewhere in the body," i.e., not where the injury actually occurred • Has to do with afferent and efferent nerve tracks, e.g., the signals have gotten crossed on the way to and from the brain • A patient with gallbladder issues may have pain in the right shoulder, but upon inspection there is no injury to the shoulder itself • Research is not yet clear on why referred pain occurs, but EMTs need to be aware of it in the field

Tearing/ Ripping Pain	• Often associated with ulcers and AAAs (abdominal aortic aneurysms)
	• Aorta spans from the heart down into the abdominal cavity and is under high pressure at all times
	• If aorta has burst or lacerated, patient will experience immense level of pain and can bleed out (internally) quickly
	• EMT may see a pulsating mass, or patient's stomach may pulsate in time with radial or carotid pulse
	• Some patients live with AAA for years and are monitored to see if it grows larger or needs surgery. Most often, a 911 call is made if the aneurysm has burst due to:
	  – Medical reason such as uncontrolled growth and breakdown of the artery tissue wall, which finally bursts
	  – Traumatic injury such as a fall or car accident

Injuries to the Genitalia

Injury to the genitalia in both males and females is extremely painful due to the high concentration of nerves in this area. Injury to this area is treated in the same way as any other wound.

Some common conditions seen in the field include:

- **Testicular torsion** is a condition where the testicle becomes twisted in the scrotum, causing severe pain. This injury is caused by strenuous activity and must be corrected in the emergency department. Care by the EMT involves application of an ice pack to relieve the pain and careful transport to minimize movement.

- **Sexual assault** victims require special handling by the emergency medical system, since EMTs are often the first responders on site.

  - The victim should be assessed by an EMT of the same gender, if possible.

  - Care should be supportive and affirming, without making unrealistic promises. Sexual assault victims are often sensitive to being touched in any way by an EMT, so it is important to keep a calm voice.

  - Remember that, unless impaired or unconscious, a patient has the right to refuse any medical procedure, so request the patient's permission to perform each and every assessment, particularly those involving the genitals.

  - Most states require medical personnel to report these events to the police, especially if the victim is a minor.

  - Be very careful to preserve any evidence of a crime, such as torn clothing and stains from blood and other fluids.

Practice Set

1. You are dispatched to a motorcycle accident on the interstate. You respond emergently and arrive on the scene 10 minutes after being dispatched. Your patient is unconscious and unresponsive to any stimuli. Your rapid assessment shows that he is breathing with ragged breaths at a rate of 16, has pulse 60 with pulse oximetry 94%. He is lying 80 feet from his motorcycle face down on the pavement. Your transport time to the trauma center is 30 minutes. How long do you have to assess and treat this patient on the scene?

   A. 10 minutes

   B. 20 minutes

   C. 30 minutes

   D. Enough time to properly treat all of the patient's injuries

2. What trauma center level provides the highest level of care with 24-hour, in-house availability of surgeons?

   A. Level 4

   B. Level 3

   C. Level 2

   D. Level 1

3. You are dispatched to a two-car accident on a rural highway. You arrive on scene and the incident commander directs you to a car that has been struck broadside by the other vehicle. There is severe damage to the driver's side of the vehicle, and the driver is lying on the front seat on her back. She is unconscious and unresponsive. She appears pale and diaphoretic with a weak, thready pulse. Her right leg is lying beneath the steering wheel at an awkward angle. She has a large scalp laceration, which is bleeding purplish blood. You are wearing suitable precautions against bloodborne pathogens. Which of the following is the next correct step in management?

   A. Gently splint the right leg with a board splint

   B. Apply a sterile dressing to the scalp laceration

   C. Perform a rapid extrication and transport priority to the trauma center

   D. Take cervical stabilization and open the airway using the modified jaw thrust

4. In the scenario in question 3, your patient is breathing at a rate of 24 times per minute and has a pulse of 80. What would be your next treatment?

   A. Assist breaths using a BVM at 20 bpm

   B. Apply a sterile dressing to the scalp laceration

   C. Perform a rapid extrication and transport priority to the trauma center

   D. Apply a cervical collar and maintain stabilization of head and neck

5. Your patient has been extricated to the truck on a backboard with full cervical stabilization. Her injuries include the right leg which has been splinted and a head wound that has been bandaged appropriately. Your assessment of the head reveals nothing remarkable but you notice a large bruise on the right side of the chest. Her blood pressure is 94/64. Which of the following is the best choice for the transport position of this patient?

    A. Raise the head of the stretcher 8–12 inches

    B. Raise the feet of the backboard 8–12 inches

    C. Keep the backboard flat

    D. Lift the left side of the backboard 2–4 inches

6. In the scenario described in question 3, your response time to the scene was 10 minutes. You now estimate it will take you 15 minutes to transport your patient to the trauma center. How many minutes should you spend triaging and treating your patient on scene?

    A. 10 minutes

    B. 20 minutes

    C. 30 minutes

    D. As long as it takes

7. Which of the following definitions best describes an avulsion?

    A. Separation of a limb or other body part from the remainder of the body

    B. A smooth or jagged cut caused by a sharp object of blunt force that tears the tissue

    C. An injury that leaves a piece of skin or other tissue partially or completely torn from the body

    D. An injury that does not break the skin but causes tissue and vascular damage under the skin

8. You respond to a fight in progress call to assist police with a possible gunshot victim. You arrive on scene wearing suitable protective equipment and the police have secured the scene. They direct you to a male in his mid-twenties, lying supine on the ground. His shirt is full of blood, and he is conscious and alert but having trouble breathing. What should be your next move?

    A. Apply a tourniquet to both arms to minimize extremity blood flow

    B. Apply an NRB mask and administer oxygen at 12 liters per minute

    C. Remove the shirt and check for wounds

    D. Place the patient on a backboard and transport immediately to the nearest trauma center

9. In the scenario in question 8, you observe a puncture wound ½ inch in diameter in the left chest 2 inches superior to the left nipple. It is actively bleeding bright red frothy blood. What is your next procedure?

    A. Apply sterile 4 × 4 gauze dressing to the wound

    B. Apply sterile occlusive dressing

    C. Apply a trauma dressing

    D. Request an ALS intercept

10. You respond to the scene of an MVA. You and your partner are assisting another ambulance crew with spinal immobilization for a patient with a suspected cervical spine injury. Which of the following EMTs will direct the movement of the patient?

    A. The most experienced EMT on the scene

    B. The highest ranking EMT on the scene

    C. The EMT holding stabilization of the head

    D. The EMT who is not actively involved in patient care

11. How do you treat an amputated finger?

    A. Transport it with the patient

    B. Secure it to the patient's hand with sterile gauze and tape

    C. Keep it cool by placing it directly on an ice pack

    D. Transport it separately in a second rescue or police car to avoid traumatizing the patient

12. Which of the following impaled objects should you remove in the field?

    A. Pencil through the cheek

    B. Fishing spear embedded in the left thigh

    C. Fence post through the abdomen

    D. Knife embedded in the chest causing a pneumothorax

13. You respond to a house explosion with fire and police. You have suitable protective equipment and the scene is secure upon your arrival. On scene you are directed to a patient with soot on his face. The patient states rather sheepishly that he was lighting his charcoal grill and, having run out of lighter fluid, poured gasoline on the charcoal and then attempted to light it, resulting in an explosion. He is conscious and alert with superficial burns to both his arms and hands and his face. What is your primary concern with this patient?

    A. Hypovolemic shock

    B. Danger of infection

    C. Airway compromise

    D. Secondary explosion

14. In the scenario in question 13, approximately what percentage of the patient's body is burned?

    A. 10%

    B. 20%

    C. 30%

    D. 40%

15. In the scenario in questions 13 and 14, in what condition is this patient considered to be?

    A. Critical

    B. Moderate

    C. Minor

    D. Fatal

16. You respond to an industrial plant for an injured worker. You respond with lights and sirens wearing suitable BSI precautions. You arrive on scene and observe a male lying atop a wire, obviously unconscious. Which of the following should be your primary concern?

    A. Airway

    B. Scene safety

    C. Burn injury

    D. Cardiac arrhythmias

17. You arrive on the scene of a motorcycle accident. The police are on scene, and you are wearing suitable BSI gear. The driver is lying supine 15 feet away from his motorcycle, which is lying on its side. He is screaming in pain, and you perform your initial assessment and rapid trauma assessment. He is conscious, alert, and oriented with no injuries other than an angulated right femur that is causing him severe pain. His vitals are BP 160/100, pulse 120, and respirations 22. Which of the following devices should you use to splint his injury?

    A. KED

    B. Traction splint

    C. Long spine board

    D. Padded board splint

18. You respond to a soccer field for an injured player. You respond emergently wearing suitable precautions. When you arrive on the scene, you are directed to the soccer field, where an 11-year-old female is conscious, alert, and oriented, lying supine in severe pain. She is clutching her left upper arm with her right hand and her shoulder is displaced to the anterior. Bystanders state she was in a collision with another player and fell to the ground. She did not lose consciousness, her vital signs are within normal limits, and the remainder of the assessment is unremarkable. What injury do you suspect?

    A. Broken humerus

    B. Broken radius

    C. Dislocated patella

    D. Dislocated shoulder

19. What does PMS stand for with regard to splinting an injury?

    A. Pulse, management, and sensory function

    B. Pulse, management, and swelling

    C. Pulse, motor, and swelling

    D. Pulse, motor, and sensory function

20. Who is responsible for directing movement of the patient when securing to a long backboard?

    A. The lead EMT on the call

    B. The EMT holding the long backboard

    C. The EMT who is logrolling the patient

    D. The EMT who is holding the cervical spine

21. You are dispatched to a man fallen off a ladder at his home. You arrive on the scene with suitable BSI precautions to find a male sitting on the floor with a blood-soaked trouser leg. He is conscious, alert, and oriented; has normal vital signs; and has no other injuries or loss of consciousness. You expose the leg by gently cutting the trouser leg away and observe that the fibula is broken and the superior end is exposed through the anterior side of the leg. It is still actively bleeding. What must you do BEFORE you splint the leg?

    A. DCAP-BTLS

    B. Feel for pedal pulse

    C. Apply a sterile dressing to the wound

    D. Irrigate the wound with sterile saline

22. In the scenario in question 21, the patient had a good pedal pulse prior to you applying the splint. Upon rechecking, it is no longer palpable, and the foot is becoming cold and cyanotic. What should you do next?

    A. Request an ALS intercept

    B. Remove the splint

    C. Expedite the transport

    D. Immobilize the patient on a backboard and transport rapidly

23. You arrive on the scene of a two-car motor vehicle accident. The incident commander directs you to the first car, which was rear-ended by the second car. The driver is alone in the vehicle and is still wearing her seat belt. She is conscious, alert, and oriented, complaining of neck pain and unable to turn her head. You and your partner are wearing appropriate BSI gear, and there is no gross hemorrhage. What should be your next move?

    A. Rapidly extricate the patient onto a long backboard

    B. Place the patient in a KED and extricate

    C. Take manual stabilization from the rear seat and apply a cervical collar

    D. Perform a modified jaw thrust

24. A patient is found lying prone on the ground, unconscious with shallow breaths at eight per minute. After performing a rapid logroll with proper cervical precautions, you find that it is difficult to manage the patient's airway without removing his full-faced motorcycle helmet. What is your next step?

    A. Remove the helmet carefully while your partner continues to hold c-spine precautions

    B. Remove the face mask only and apply an NRB at 15 lpm

    C. Remove the helmet while your partner hooks up a BVM to the oxygen cylinder

    D. Perform a head-tilt, chin-lift with the helmet in place and see if his breathing improves

25. You are dispatched to a home under construction for a man fallen off a roof. Your patient is a roofer who walked off the roof and fell approximately 20 feet to the ground. He is conscious but dazed. He has an airway, his respiratory rate is 14, and his pulse is 72. There is no gross hemorrhage or sign of any bleeding. Your partner takes manual stabilization of the head and neck while you perform a rapid trauma assessment, which is negative for any potentially broken bones. You apply a cervical collar and logroll him onto a backboard and secure him. En route to the trauma center, you expose the patient by cutting off his clothes, and your focused exam is negative; however, when you push against his feet, he complains of pain in the back of his neck. What injury should you suspect?

    A. Ruptured spleen

    B. Broken femur

    C. Fractured cervical vertebra

    D. Fractured skull

26. You respond to the local construction site for a man with an abdominal injury. After taking proper BSI precautions, you find what appears to be parts of his intestines coming out of a large laceration to his lower abdomen. He is tachypneic, anxious, and pale in color. What is your next step?

    A. Call for ALS while you attempt to calm the patient down

    B. Place him on a NC at 8 lpm

    C. Cover the intestines with a moist sterile dressing and secure on four sides with tape

    D. Attempt to place the intestines back inside with gloved hands and secure with a moist, sterile dressing

Answers and Explanations

1. A

You may be tempted to take the 60 minutes of the "golden hour," subtract the 10 minute response time and the 30 minute hospital transport time, and arrive at 20 minutes, but that does not factor in the amount of time that transpired before you were dispatched. This will be the sum of the minutes spent until someone finds the patient, dials, and is connected to the dispatch center, and the lag time while dispatch processes the incoming information and dispatches your unit. This amount of time is a variable and is dependent on a number of factors. In addition, once you arrive at the trauma center, medical personnel will triage the patient and stabilize him in the emergency department before sending him to the operating suite, which will add more minutes. (D) may sound logically correct, but if you properly treat all of these injuries on the scene you will definitely exceed the "golden hour."

2. D

The main difference between level 1 and level 2 trauma centers is that level 2 may have 24-hour availability of general surgeons but they may not necessarily be in-house.

3. D

The temptation is always to treat the most noticeable condition first, such as the active bleeding or the obvious fracture. However, you first and foremost must be concerned with the patient's survival; without an airway, she will be dead in minutes. In addition, the patient's cervical spine must be stabilized prior to any other treatments to minimize the danger of damaging the spinal cord. (D) takes care of both those things and must be the priority in this scenario.

4. D

There is no indication that a rapid extrication is needed. There is a temptation is to treat the obvious head wound, but since the bleeding is purplish and non-pulsing, it is probably venous and can be controlled once your patient is better stabilized and extricated.

5. C

While some may argue that (B) is correct if shock is suspected, studies and research suggest that we move away from the Trendelenburg position when treating shock. (A) is incorrect as we do not lift the head of the patient, while (D) is used to treat supine hypotensive syndrome. Choice (C) is correct, ie, keep the backboard flat.

6. A

The correct answer is 10 minutes. Twenty minutes will still be under the 1 hour guide, but does not take into account discovery and notification time, nor triage time at the hospital. Thirty minutes will obviously put you over the 1 hour, as would the impossible luxury of "taking as long as you like." This scene is managed by quickly performing the procedures necessary to save the patient's life and packaging her for transport. Further assessments and treatments may be accomplished en route.

7. C

An avulsion is partial or complete tearing of a piece of skin. (A) is an amputation, (B) is a laceration, and (D) is a contusion.

8. C

You need to visualize what you're dealing with to be able to intervene properly. Applying a tourniquet to minimize extremity blood flow is not an acceptable procedure for this injury. You may well want to administer supplemental oxygen after you've done a proper assessment, but the assessment is the important thing at this stage.

9. B

The correct next procedure is to apply a sterile occlusive dressing. (A) and (C) will do nothing to seal the opening in the pleural space that air is escaping from, which is what is causing the frothy blood. The danger here is that this patient will develop a tension pneumothorax or hemothorax. You may request an ALS intercept to assist with advanced life support measures; however, you would do this after you have taken care of the life-threatening conditions, such as the gross hemorrhage.

10. C

The EMT holding stabilization of the head is always responsible for directing the movement of the patient.

11. A

The amputated extremity should be wrapped in a sterile wet dressing, placed in a cool container, and transported with the patient to the appropriate facility. Attempting to secure it to the patient's hand with gauze and tape will only delay transport and not have any long-term benefit. Placing it directly on an ice pack could cause it to freeze and the tissue to die. There is no reason to transport it separately either.

12. A

The correct answer is (A), because a pencil through the cheek will interfere with respiration. The other answers will not impede the airway and should be left for the emergency department to deal with.

13. C

The correct answer is airway compromise. The nature of the explosion and the fact that his face is burned gives him a high probability that he inhaled the flame and smoke from the explosion. The danger of infection is less problematic than the risk of his airway swelling shut. A secondary explosion has hopefully been minimized by the fire department's securing of the scene.

14. B

Using the rule of nines, each arm counts for 9% for a total of 18. The whole head is 9%, but in this case, only the face is involved and counts for 4.5%. This gives a total of 22.5%, and answer choice (B) is the closest.

15. A

This is a critical patient because of the danger of airway compromise due to burns to his face. The patient could also be considered critical simply because two entire body parts, the arms, are involved. Some test takers may incorrectly answer "moderate" because they base their answer only by the percentage of body area affected, which is less than the 50% necessary for this burn to be considered critical if there were no other factors to consider.

16. B

The correct answer is scene safety. All of the other answer choices become concerns once you have determined that the patient is not being energized by the wire he is lying across.

17. B

While any of the devices listed may be used, the traction splint is the preferred device for this injury.

18. D

It is important to read the question and get a picture of what is being described. You could stop with the upper arm and deduce that the correct answer is the broken humerus, but the anterior displacement of the shoulder is the key that this is a dislocation or fracture of the shoulder joint.

19. D

To test for motor movement, you would ask the patient to wiggle their toes/finger and grip the EMT's fingers. Sensory function is tested by asking which finger or toe the EMT is touching or if they feel pain when performing any commands.

20. D

The correct answer is (D) due to the importance of maintaining as straight a spine as possible. Due to this significance, they must make sure that all team members know when to start and stop a transfer move.

21. C

This is a combination of an open wound and a fracture, and both must be treated. You will already have done DCAP-BTLS to find this, and while you will want to check for a pedal pulse the key here is that the wound is still actively bleeding. Irrigation of the wound may or may not be advisable due to a number of conditions, which is why (C) is the best answer.

22. B

In applying the splint, you may have occluded an artery supplying blood to the foot. The other answers are all possibilities, but you have to correct the problem that was caused by applying the splint too tightly or incorrectly.

23. C

The patient is talking to you, so you know that there is an airway and that the patient is breathing. Before extricating her from the vehicle, your next priority is to secure the head and neck. Whether either a long or short backboard is used, the neck must be secured in a properly sized c-collar. There is no indication for a jaw thrust to be used in this scenario.

24. A

The key to this question is that the patient is found originally laying prone and breathing with an inadequate rate and depth. Because we are not given information as to how the patient ended up in this scenario, (A) is the safest way to manage this patient. (D) would only be used if cervical spine injury can be ruled out, and in this scenario it would be unsafe to do so. (B) and (C) deal with airway management, but one EMT needs to hold onto the cervical spine, making (C) incorrect. (B) only removes part of the helmet, and an NRB is not appropriate for this type of aggressive airway management.

25. C

Pain to the neck as you are applying pressure to the soles of the feet indicates some type of pressure to the spinal cord. All of the other injuries are possible given the MOI, however there is nothing in the question to indicate that any of these are the correct answer.

26. C

While (A) is definitely a good idea, (C) is the correct answer here, as this is an emergent situation where the intestines must remain moist and secured. This patient needs urgent surgical attention, and if the proper facility is closer than ALS interception do not delay transport. Never attempt (D).

CHAPTER 8

Pediatrics

Topics Discussed

- Pediatric Assessment Considerations
- ABCs in the Pediatric Patient
- Special Conditions and Scenarios
- Child Abuse and Neglect
- Trauma Equipment
- Transport Considerations

Pediatrics is a generalized term that ranges from infants to young adults aged 18. It is important to realize that people in this age bracket are not just little adults. There are very real differences in pediatric anatomy and physiology, as well as psychological and sociological factors, which make the study of pediatrics in the prehospital setting a true specialty. In addition, the EMT must be prepared to deal with the caregivers of this group, who will present another dimension to the issue of providing quality care to the younger patient.

Assessment

In pediatrics more than in adult assessment, an EMT's initial impression of the patient's condition as the scene is first observed is most important. A child who is actually sick looks sick.

Special concerns in the pediatric population include epiglottitis and croup. The assessment and intervention protocols for these special conditions are state-specific; some states (but not all) allow an EMT to administer epinephrine via nebulizer if croup or epiglottitis is suspected, with permission from medical control.

Children often lack an understanding of the structure and function of the human body or have an incorrect understanding of the role that organs play. Be sure to explain in very simple terms what is going on with an injury.

Use the following guidelines for pediatric assessment:

- When you approach the child, be gentle and kind. Sick children have a very real fear of being sick, or even dying. Your presence must be reassuring and not threatening.

- Try to connect with the child's emotions. It helps to get down to the child's eye level or sit alongside on the ground.
- To assess the child's mental status, announce your presence as you would with an adult and gauge the child's response to voice, touch, or painful stimuli. You must ascertain whether the child's reaction to your (EMS) presence is normal for a child of that age. It is a normal reaction, for example, for a toddler to cry as you approach, as a child this age will often cry at the approach of a uniformed stranger.
- To do the physical exam, start at the feet and work up toward the head.

When performing interventions and collecting vital signs, it is important that the devices used are properly sized for the size of the patient.

- **Broselow tape**: color-coded tape measure, standardized and used worldwide for pediatric emergencies
  - Provides a rapid estimate of the child's weight based on body length
  - Allows EMS to determine proper dosing, sizing for airway equipment, and level of shock voltage when using a defibrillator
  - Tape is marked with colors and a weight (in kilograms, because certain medications are weight-based in the ALS level of care)
- **Handtevy method**: tool that uses both age and length to assess amount of medication needed in pediatric emergencies
  - Uses both a tape with prewritten dosages and the provider's hands to "count"
  - Associates five age categories (ages 1, 3, 5, 7, and 9) with their corresponding weight (in kilograms) via a finger-counting method on the hand
- **Blood pressure cuffs**, **pulse oximeter probes**, **OPA/NPAs**, and even the **bell of a stethoscope** all come in pediatric sizes. An adult size in any of these devices will not give an accurate reading on children.

Remember that "normal" vital signs are different for children than for adults. Infants, for example, will have normal respiratory rates in the 40s, which would call for positive pressure ventilation support in the adult population.

To convert pounds to kilograms, use the following formula:

$$\text{Number of kilograms (kg)} = \frac{\text{Number of pounds (lb)}}{2.2046}$$

While the exam is not likely to include calculation questions about dosage, you may be asked once you are on the job if you know how much a child weighs. Therefore, it is a good idea to know how to convert kilograms to pounds.

A big difference between adult and pediatric assessment is that the **physical exam begins at the feet and works upward toward the head**. Touching a child's head, especially among preschoolers, can increase anxiety, and it is better to have completed the rest of the body before this occurs.

Psychological and Social Factors

In performing assessment on a pediatric patient, the EMT must take into consideration psychological and sociological factors characteristic of this population.

- **Toddlers and preschoolers** generally will have a fear of separation from their parents or caregivers and may be very suspicious of strangers. They may rebel at being touched or examined by strangers and will be fearful of masks and needles. If one is available, a parent is the best person to provide patient history, as the child may be unable to communicate important medical history and medication use. It is helpful to have a stuffed animal or use parents as "examples" to show the patient what you want to do, and they will be more willing to allow assessment.
- **School-age children and adolescents** will be more social and open to EMT intervention since they have usually begun social interaction in the school setting.
- **Older adolescents** may have to be assessed privately, since they might want to keep issues such as sexual activity and substance abuse hidden from their parents.

Subsets of the pediatric population:

- **Neonates**: age of birth–4 weeks
- **Infants**: age 4 weeks–1 year
- **Toddlers**: age 1–3 years
- **Preschoolers**: age 3–6 years
- **School-age children**: age 6–10 years
- **Adolescents**: age 11–21 years (updated in 2017 by the American Academy of Pediatrics)

Age 21 is the typical cut-off for pediatric patient care, except when some chronic pediatric illnesses extend longer.

Physical Factors

The first thing to note with neonates and infants is that they cannot support their necks and heads on their own, so they must always be held in such a way that supports their neck/head. In addition, the differences in pediatric airway anatomy present real concerns to the EMT.

- Neonates and infants have a larger tongue and smaller trachea than adults.
- The epiglottis of neonates and infants is located much higher in the airway than it is in adults.
- The heads of younger children are proportionally larger than those of older children and adults, which can present special problems in the case of trauma.

Children do not typically live alone, and at a young age are not able to make their own decisions. Therefore, any EMS call involving a pediatric patient will require attention to both the child and the parent/caregiver.

- Children are very perceptive and will quickly pick up on the EMT's confidence or uncertainty. Project a knowledgeable, confident, take-charge approach.
- Parents may have received specialized training for their child's medical care and can thus be an important resource.
- Children who are seriously injured or ill are almost always comforted by the presence of a parent or caregiver. (Exceptions include a parent/caregiver who is abusing the child.) The general rule is that a **calm parent will yield a calm child** (similarly, an anxious parent will yield an anxious child), so help to make that happen. If the parent is calm and can convey that calmness to the child, that will go a long way in the child's compliance. Options include:
  - Have the parent secured on the bench seat in plain view of the secured child during transport, as being able to see the caregiver will be calming
  - Have the parent ride up front with you

Physiological Factors

Compared with adults, pediatric vital signs tend to skew higher the younger the child is. As the child begins to age, the main vital signs of respiratory rate, pulse, and blood pressure will begin to move toward what they will be for most of adulthood.

In general, children have a faster heartbeat, faster respiratory rate, and lower blood pressure than adults.

Table 8.1 *Pediatric Vital Signs*

Age	Respiratory Rate	Pulse	Systolic Blood Pressure
Newborn/Neonate (age birth to 1 month)	30–50 beats per min	120–160 beats per min	50–70 mm Hg
Infant (age 1–12 months)	20–30 beats per min	80–140 beats per min	70–100 mm Hg
Toddler (age 1–3 years)	20–30 beats per min	80–130 beats per min	80–110 mm Hg
Preschool (age 3–5 years)	20–30 beats per min	80–120 beats per min	80–110 mm Hg
School-age (age 6–10 years)	20–30 beats per min	70–110 beats per min	80–120 mm Hg
Adolescent (age 11+ years)	12–20 beats per min	55–105 beats per min	110–120 mm Hg

Knowing the normal ranges for each age group can help the EMT recognize whether a child is in distress. If an adult is breathing 30 times per minute, that would be considered tachypneic; however, in a child age 2, that would be considered normal.

Airway, Breathing, and Circulation

As with an adult, the ABCs of a child must be assessed and corrected first, before proceeding with treatment. Note two things:

- Equipment is available that is specifically sized for the pediatric population. Do not use adult equipment on children unless absolutely needed.

- Children are not able to compensate as long as adults, so time is of the essence in treatment for a very sick child.

Airway

Neonates and infants are nose-breathers, so suctioning the nose with a bulb syringe will often relieve a child who is having trouble breathing. When you secure the airway, be careful not to hypoextend or hyperextend the neck and kink the very small airway. A small towel/blanket placed underneath the child's shoulders can help keep the head tilted at a more neutral position than would the full head-chin lift technique used with adults.

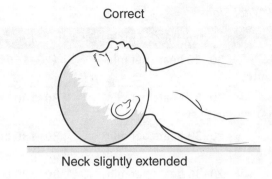

Correct

Neck slightly extended

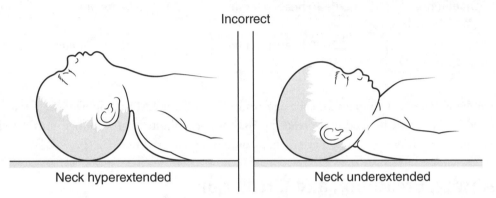

Incorrect

Neck hyperextended

Neck underextended

Figure 8.1 *Pediatric Airway Positioning*

When inserting an oropharyngeal or nasopharyngeal airway or when preparing to suction, the proper method of measuring the device is critical. Inserting an oral airway in a pediatric patient is done only in the anatomical position, using a tongue depressor or laryngoscope blade to push the tongue out of the way. If inserting a nasal airway, use lubrication to ease insertion.

The method for measuring is similar to that for an adult, with minor differences and a smaller device. With an **OPA**, measure from the corner of mouth to the tip of the earlobe. With an **NPA**, measure from the nare to the angle of mandible.

Breathing

Breathing is measured both for rate and quality, and circulation is checked. It is important to begin oxygen therapy immediately for all children in respiratory distress. If there is severe respiratory distress, provide for assistance in ventilation.

Signs of severe respiratory distress are as follows:

- Rates outside of the normal range
- Presence of cyanosis
- Respiratory distress with poor muscle tone
- See-saw breathing
- Accessory muscles, especially noticeable in the lateral rib view

Oxygen Therapy

Some services carry masks in pediatric-friendly designs, such as dragons and panda bears. If your service doesn't have these, they are required to at least have pediatric-sized nasal cannulas (NC) and non-rebreather masks (NRB). There are also appropriately sized BVMs to deliver more accurate tidal volumes. It is up to the EMT to measure and utilize each piece of equipment properly.

- Neonates and infants will rarely accept an NC or NRB, so administer oxygen therapy with oxygen tubing (called **blow-by oxygenation**).
  - Hold oxygen tubing 2 inches away from the nose and mouth, and simply flow the oxygen over that area.
  - Alternatively, hold a paper cup (also 2 inches away) and blow the oxygen into the cup, creating an oxygen reservoir.
- Older children are much more likely to accept an NC or NRB. Place it as you would for an adult.

In a team-based resuscitation effort, the ratio of compressions to breaths should be 15:2 for children, which allows the rescuer to deliver breaths using a BVM at a rate of 20–30 breaths per minute. The volume delivered is also less than when ventilating an adult, so be sure to not overinflate the lungs and stop squeezing the BVM when you see chest rise.

Circulation

Checking circulation involves verification of a pulse, skin color and condition, capillary refill, and if any major bleeds are present.

The absence of pulses is the indication to begin CPR, and the rate and method must be correct for the age of the child.

- Single rescuer CPR is a ratio of compressions to breath of 30:2.
- Two or more rescuer CPR changes the ratio to 15:2.
- Per AHA standards, if an infant is found to have a pulse <60 bpm, compressions are to be started at the appropriate ratio.

In infants, pulse is checked on the brachial artery in the upper arm. In children and teen-agers, pulse is checked on the carotid or radial artery.

Special Conditions

Seizures

High core body temperatures resulting from infection may cause pediatric seizures. These seizures are referred to as **febrile seizures**. A febrile seizure can be confirmed by checking the patient's forehead for a higher-than-normal temperature. If skin temperature is normal or below normal, then the cause of the seizure may be hypoxia, poisoning, trauma, hypoglycemia, or some other cause.

The patient's seizure history and medications should be determined. The patient's airway must be secured, the patient transported on his or her side, and oxygen therapy initiated. If the patient feels warm to the touch, a cool, damp towel applied to the head may be effective in lowering the body temperature enough to cancel the seizure. Remember that following a seizure, the patient will be postictal for a period of time.

Altered Mental Status

This condition may be caused by a variety of conditions, including seizures, hypoglycemia, poisoning, trauma, hypoxia, and shock.

The treatment regimen is the same as with the adult population: secure the airway, administer oxygen, administer medication per local protocol, and transport to an appropriate hospital—ideally a pediatric-specific emergency department.

Poisoning

Since children are curious, poisoning is a major cause of visits to the emergency department. If you suspect poisoning or overdose you must make an effort while still on scene to locate the container that holds the substance ingested by the child, as this will give important information as to antidotes and treatment.

If the patient is still responsive, contact medical control to check if activated charcoal may be administered in accordance with local protocols. Activated charcoal is an absorbent that will help prevent the toxin from being further absorbed into the bloodstream.

If the patient is unconscious, nothing may be given by mouth, as this may cause choking and an occluded airway. Maintain the airway, administer oxygen, and transport priority.

Shock (Hypoperfusion)

In the pediatric population, unlike the adult population, shock is rarely a cardiac event, but it is usually brought on by dehydration secondary to a variety of illnesses. Dehydration will usually coincide with hypoperfusion, which is more problematic since young children have a much lower blood supply than adults to begin with. Low blood pressure in a pediatric patient is a late sign of shock and requires a more aggressive approach to treatment than in an adult. In infants and toddlers, decreased urine output and dry crying (crying without tears) are good indicators of dehydration.

Shock in children calls for rapid transport with anti-shock measures as per the local protocols, including the use of an ALS intercept if indicated. These measures routinely include keeping the patient warm, administering oxygen, and rapidly transporting to an appropriate facility.

Near Drowning

A cold, lifeless appearance of a near-drowning victim requires aggressive resuscitation efforts by EMS personnel and rapid transport to a pediatric trauma center. Just because someone is cold to the touch and unresponsive does not mean they are deceased, especially if only a short amount of time has passed.

Good ventilation technique has resulted in the resuscitation of many children thought to be dead from near drowning in cold water.

Respiratory distress is also a possibility with children who have suffered a near-drowning experience but were breathing fine after the event. Any victim of a near drowning should be transported to a pediatric emergency department for evaluation, if available.

Child Abuse and Neglect

Abuse is when improper or excessive action has caused harm or injury to someone. Abuse may be physical, psychological, or emotional in nature. **Neglect** is insufficient attention or respect to someone with a claim to that attention.

While these concepts can be subjective, the EMT must always err on the side of the patient: **if there is any suspicion of abuse or neglect, it must be reported to the proper authorities**. Failure to report, in many jurisdictions, is a crime in itself and can subject the EMT to criminal and civil penalties. Some guidelines include:

- Infant left in a locked auto without any supervision (**obvious neglect**)
- EMS intervention to a house where there is no adult present and small children are left alone (**very suspicious but not clear-cut neglect**; explore why this has occurred)
- Multiple EMS interventions to the same address or same patient (**very suspicious**)
- Unexplained bruises, injuries inconsistent with the explanation, conflicting stories of how the injury occurred, fresh burns, fear in the face of the child, and dismissiveness by the parents (**very suspicious**)
- Child who appears malnourished, unsafe, or to be living in unhealthy living conditions or with untreated chronic illnesses (**very suspicious and could be considered both neglect and abuse**)
- Infant who presents with CNS deficiencies (**suspicious for shaken baby syndrome**, in which violent shaking has damaged the spinal cord)
  - Often results in death of the infant.
  - Your run report must be clear and concise about the facts of the call, to assist authorities in the proper disposition of the situation.

If you suspect abuse or neglect, it is not your job to accuse the parents or caregivers. Your main focus is to care for the patient.

- You will certainly need to report your suspicions (and supporting evidence) to the authorities, usually the local police, but that is done later.
- Make sure you report this directly by either online form, telephone report, or orally to appropriate personnel, i.e., do not rely on anyone else to communicate the information. In many states, EMS staff are considered "mandatory reporters," and they must fill out appropriate paperwork besides their PCR. This is necessary, since this agency's interaction with the parent and patient is critical for getting the child appropriate help.

- You should also share this information with the receiving facility to ensure that the patient receives proper treatment.
- Lastly, some states require that their children's health and safety agencies be notified of suspected abuse or neglect. Each state has a different reporting system, and you must follow its procedure.

Sudden Infant Death Syndrome (SIDS)

There are few calls that are more traumatic in EMS than "child not breathing." SIDS is a condition in which a previously healthy infant is found in the crib not breathing, and the postmortem can find no cause for the death. It is important to remember that the patients in these calls include the parents of the child, and proper care means that someone must intervene with them, even if it requires calling for more personnel to the scene or a second rescue.

Many states require that resuscitation efforts be undertaken, even in the presence of biological death indicators such as rigor mortis and postmortem lividity, if for no other reason than to assure the parents that everything possible has been done for their child. While nothing will compensate for the loss of a child, a professional, assuring demeanor toward the parents may provide a small measure of comfort in this traumatic situation.

Special Needs Infants and Children

Many infants and children with chronic conditions are cared for at home by their parents and visiting health care workers. Emergencies in this population are common, and 911 is often called. EMS is usually the service to respond and intervene.

While EMT courses rarely go into detail on the emergency treatment of children with special needs, the well-versed EMT tries to keep abreast of these procedures so that interventions are correct.

Common conditions among this population include:

- **Child who has had a tracheostomy tube surgically implanted in the trachea**
  - Tracheostomy tubes may become plugged with mucus, which may cause the child to present with difficulty breathing. Suction the tubes in the same manner as you would suction fluid from the oropharynx.
  - Do not suction for more than 5 seconds at a time, and administer oxygen to the tube between suctioning attempts.
  - In the event of respiratory failure, use the tube to administer positive pressure ventilation directly to the trachea, while blocking the nose and mouth. Yankauer tips do not often fit, so use a soft French catheter instead.
  - If a tube becomes dislodged or is removed by the patient, the stoma or opening can be used to ventilate and may have to be suctioned, especially if bleeding is present because of the removal of the tube.

- Do not attempt to replace a tracheostomy tube that has been removed or dislodged. Instead, transport the child to the nearest pediatric care facility.

- Look for signs of infection such as swelling and redness around the site.

- **Child who is in chronic respiratory failure, possibly connected to a home ventilator**

  - Parents are usually well instructed in the use of a home ventilator and often have a backup in place.

  - If you are called and none of the devices will operate properly, be prepared to manually ventilate the patient with an oxygen-supplied bag-valve mask and transport priority to the nearest facility.

- **Central IV lines** have been placed in the larger veins of the torso in order to supply medication that is needed on a regular basis.

  - If you encounter complications from these lines, transport the patient to a pediatric hospital for proper management.

  - En route, support the airway, assist in respiration, and control any bleeding.

- **Gastrostomy tubes** are implanted directly into the stomach for children who cannot be fed by mouth.

  - If you see that the tubes have become dislodged or plugged and the parents have not been trained in their reinsertion, transport the patient to a pediatric hospital for proper management.

  - En route, support the breathing.

- **Shunts** are tubes that are placed inside the skull to divert excess fluid to the stomach or to a reservoir on the side of the neck.

  - If this device fails, the patient will present with signs of brain injury, such as change in mental status, seizures, nausea, vomiting, and loss of motor control.

  - If you find that the shunt has failed, transport the patient to the nearest facility right away.

  - En route, support the airway and assist in respiration.

  - This is a severe condition.

- **Autism and sensory disorders**

  - Children on the autism spectrum range from low to high functioning. Many, but not all, are nonverbal and sensitive to changes in their environment (including EMS arrival). If they are older, speak with them in age-appropriate language and give them respect and time to answer your questions.

  - Oftentimes, the caregiver is the "gateway" into gaining trust to allow the provider to do an assessment.

  - Aim to make the child as comfortable as possible by explaining everything you are doing (include the caregiver as well).

  - Use lights and sirens cautiously, as they may make certain children more reactive or exacerbate symptoms.

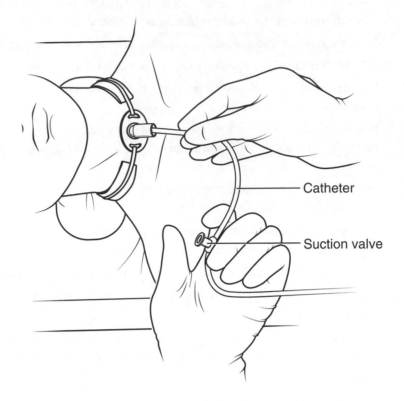

Figure 8.2 *Tracheostomy Tube with Suction*

Trauma

Trauma, especially motor vehicle trauma, is the number one cause of death in the pediatric population. Head injuries and internal organ injuries are common, while bone injuries are less common.

- **Head injuries** are common because a child's head is proportionally larger than the rest of the body.
- **Organ injuries** are common because the pliability of the child's bones means that the internal organs are not well protected (unlike adults, whose stronger bones provide more protection to the internal organs).
- **Bone injuries** are less common because the pliability of the child's bones means they are less likely to be fractured from blunt-force trauma.

Assessment of pediatric trauma is the same as for adults, except that you should begin the physical exam at the feet and work toward the head (in the case of a conscious patient).

Treatment of pediatric trauma is the same as for adults, although pediatric-specific equipment must be used to protect the child as much as possible. Examples of equipment that is available in pediatric sizes include:

- Traction splints
- Immobilization board
- C-collars
- Padded board splints

When transporting a child, use a pediatric-specific harness. (There are several types available, so know which one your service uses.) A transporting harness mimics a car seat and is a much safer transport option for children.

Use a car seat attached to the stretcher only as a last resort.

When transporting a child, it is imperative that the child **not ride on the caregiver's lap** while secured to the stretcher. Many injuries have occurred in this scenario.

Practice Set

1. A pediatric patient who is 4 years old is categorized as a

    A. neonate.
    B. infant.
    C. toddler.
    D. preschooler.

2. An adolescent is defined as being in which age range?

    A. 6–12 years old
    B. 11–21 years old
    C. 13–18 years old
    D. 10–15 years old

3. The airway of an infant is proportionally _____ the airway of an adolescent.

    A. smaller than
    B. larger than
    C. the same size as
    D. inverse to

4. A 6-month-old infant presents with difficulty breathing. Which characteristic of this child may account for this?

    A. Proportionally larger head
    B. Proportionally larger trachea
    C. Obligatory nose-breather
    D. Higher respiratory rate

5. Which piece of equipment would be beneficial in treating the patient in question 4?

    A. Non-rebreather mask
    B. Vacuum suction unit
    C. Bulb syringe
    D. Magill forceps

6. Which set of the vital signs listed below are considered normal for a neonate?

    A. Pulse 140, respirations 40
    B. Pulse 140, respirations 80
    C. Pulse 80, respirations 40
    D. Pulse 80, respirations 60

7. While performing the physical assessment on a 3-year-old who fell off a wall and whose parents are not yet on scene, you begin to palpate his neck. He begins to cry and tries to pull himself away from you. This action indicates which of the following?

    A. Possible child abuse
    B. Possible carotid-artery bruise
    C. Possible pneumothorax
    D. Possible cerebrovascular accident

8. Which of the following techniques should be used to open the airway of a 1-year-old in respiratory arrest?

    A. Head-tilt, chin-lift
    B. Modified jaw thrust
    C. Heimlich maneuver
    D. Valsalva maneuver

9. Which of the following should NOT be used to administer oxygen to a pediatric patient?

    A. Pediatric face mask
    B. Paper cup and oxygen tubing
    C. Blow-by technique
    D. Oxygen-powered manual respirator

10. You should begin the physical examination of a pediatric patient at the

    A. head.
    B. shoulders.
    C. buttocks.
    D. feet.

11. The pulse that should be checked on an infant is located at the

    A. radial artery.
    B. brachial artery.
    C. carotid artery.
    D. femoral artery.

12. The most common cause of seizures in the pediatric population is

    A. poisoning.
    B. hypoxia.
    C. fever.
    D. epilepsy.

13. SIDS stands for

    A. Sudden Idiopathic Dyspnea Syndrome.
    B. Shaken Infant Death Syndrome.
    C. Sudden Infant Development Syndrome.
    D. Sudden Infant Death Syndrome.

14. Which of the following needs to be treated in a SIDS situation?

    A. The infant
    B. The parents
    C. The EMS responders
    D. All of the above

15. In examining a 7-year-old for a possible broken arm, you notice that his legs are covered with bruises. He cannot explain how they got there and appears withdrawn and defensive. You feel that this patient may be at risk for or a victim of child abuse. To whom should you report this?

    A. The parents
    B. The social worker at the receiving medical facility
    C. The state agency charged with child protection
    D. The media

Answers and Explanations

1. D

A 4-year-old is a preschooler. Neonates are 1 day to 4 weeks old; infants, 4 weeks to 1 year old; and toddlers, 1 to 3 years old.

2. B

You have to read this question and all of the answers carefully. The American Pediatric Association classifies adolescence as being between 11–21 years of age. Each answer contains partially correct ranges, but (B) is the most correct.

3. A

The infant's airway is proportionally smaller than that of the adolescent. Please note the presence of the key word *proportionally*.

4. C

Since neonates and infants are obligatory nose-breathers, the accumulation of mucus in the nasopharynx would cause dyspnea. The size of the head has nothing to do with breathing. Pediatric patients have a relatively smaller trachea, making (B) incorrect. (D), while having to do with respirations, would not be directly related to causing dyspnea.

5. C

A bulb syringe is used to apply gentle suction and clear the nasal passages of mucus, which will facilitate breathing. A non-rebreather mask (A) is used for high-flow oxygen administration, a vacuum suction unit (B) is too powerful to be used on a 6-month-old, and Magill forceps (D) are used to remove foreign bodies from the oropharynx and trachea.

6. A

Normal pulses for a newborn are in a range from 100–180. Respiratory rates are in a range of 30–60. If you were sure of the pulse range, you could eliminate the last two answers and focus on (A) or (B).

7. B

A carotid artery bruise would be painful to the touch and would increase the child's anxiety level. Child abuse is a tempting answer, except that the patient's response is fairly normal given the patient's age; he should be suspicious of strangers. There is nothing in the question that would indicate a pneumothorax (C) or CVA (D).

8. A

The correct answer is (A) but with precautions to not hyper- or hypoextend the child's neck so that the airway is not occluded. (B) would be appropriate if spinal injury were suspected, but it is not in this scenario. The Heimlich maneuver (C) is used to dislodge the airway obstruction of an adult, and the Valsalva maneuver (D) is performed on patients with supraventricular tachycardia.

9. D

(A), (B), and (C) are all methods of pediatric oxygen delivery. The manual oxygen-powered respirator should not be used in the pediatric population due to the risk of lung rupture from over-pressure.

10. D

Starting at the feet is the reverse of the physical examination technique for an adult. The reason for starting at the feet is that when you begin to examine the head, the anxiety level of the child will increase. If you have already examined the rest of the body, you will be in a good position to finish quickly and with a minimum of anxiety.

11. B

The brachial artery is the most accessible at this age.

12. C

While the other answer choices are all causes of seizures as well, most pediatric seizures are caused by high core temperatures.

13. D

Be sure to read the question and all of the answers before selecting one. Many people will answer (C) and not even read (D), simply because the first two words are part of the correct answer. But (D) is the correct answer.

14. D

While your primary concern will be the infant in cardiopulmonary arrest, the parents will be anxious and concerned and need to be attended to as well. Since we know this is a SIDS case, the outcome is not in question, and the EMS responders will need to be debriefed for critical incident stress as well.

15. C

As the person who is often first on scene and is the one to have the suspicions, the EMT is required in many states to notify the state agency responsible for child protection. It is not appropriate to notify the parents, as they may be the cause of the abuse. The social worker could be notified, but it is more important for the EMT to notify the nurse or physician caring for the patient. For obvious reasons, the media is not the appropriate agency to notify.

CHAPTER 9

Ambulance Operations

Topics Discussed

- **Preparation**
- **The Truck Check**
- **Dispatch**
- **En Route to the Scene**
- **Arrival on Scene**
- **En Route to the Receiving Facility**
- **At the Receiving Facility**
- **Postrun**
- **Air Medical Considerations**
- **Radio Communications**
- **Special Situations**

All professional-grade EMTs know that failure to plan is planning to fail. Every successful call depends on being physically and emotionally prepared to face the stresses of sudden illness, injury, hysteria, chaos, and even death. In addition, each on-duty EMT must be dressed in the uniform prescribed by the service. A professional appearance is vital if the EMT is to be taken seriously as a medical provider.

Preparing for a Call

In preparation for a call, there are two things that need be completed: equipment check and truck check.

Depending on your service, you may have only one partner or a multiple-person crew. The checks should be divided equally among all members. (If on an ALS unit, the paramedic will likely check her own equipment/drug box, while the EMT will check everything else.)

Whichever way the work is divided up, the following things must be completed *prior to* your first call.

Equipment Check

Apart from being physically ready for an emergency call, it is important to check your equipment to make sure all items are ready to go. You might get a standardized checklist from your service, but it will soon become second nature to know what equipment should and should not be on your truck. Many EMS providers can do the checklist from memory, but you may also be required to submit a physical checklist to your supervisor for each shift.

The following is a list of basic items that all EMS professionals should check at the beginning of each shift, but be aware this is not comprehensive:

- Check that medications are full and not expired
- Check that oxygen tanks as well as regulators are full and in working condition
- Restock any supplies that may not have been restocked by previous crew
- Make sure there are various sizes and adequate amounts of PPE available for crew
- Verify there are enough cleaning supplies on the unit for cleaning after each call
- Verify street maps or GPS machines are working correctly
- Check that protocols are up-to-date and you are informed of any changes
- If your service still uses paper forms, check that you have the proper paperwork in adequate amounts
- If your service uses ePCRs, make sure the computer is charged and has a charging cable
- Confirm that all radio equipment and company phones are charged and working

While not common, it has happened that EMTs have arrived on scene with empty oxygen bottles and dead batteries in their AEDs. Make sure that checking your equipment becomes an automatic part of your routine.

A basic life-support EMS unit must have at least two licensed/certified EMTs on board: one to drive and one to perform patient care. It is common procedure throughout a shift that the two EMTs rotate duties. In the event of a serious call, it is preferable for two licensed/certified EMTs to be in the patient-care compartment, while a certified driver takes over the operation of the unit.

If the EMT is part of an ALS unit, there will be a minimum of one EMT and one paramedic on board. In systems that have multiple personnel on a unit, patient care typically falls to the paramedic first who then will complete an assessment and determine what level of care the patient requires.

Regardless of how many people are on the unit, the EMT is a vital part of the team; that includes sharing responsibilities that are not always patient-care related, such as stocking, restocking, navigation, and radio or computer operations.

Truck Check

At the beginning of your shift, you will be briefed by the personnel going off duty as to the truck and the condition of supplies. At that point you should begin your truck check, as follows:

Table 9.1 *Truck Check Components*

Area to Check	Components
Physical Truck Components	• Fluid levels are adequate (i.e., oil, windshield fluid, brake fluid) • Emergency lights are operational • Tires are inflated adequately • Sirens are in working order • Doors lock and unlock properly • Seat belts are in working order • Truck exterior is washed and cleaned
Medical Supplies	• Medications are not expired • Administration units are intact, i.e., lancets for glucose monitoring, nasal atomizers (if available), syringes for drawing up medications • Bandaging supplies are stocked in proper amounts • PPE supplies are available for every crew member

Medical Equipment	• Stretcher is in working order and cleaned
	• Batteries are charged and in operating order for equipment, such as:
	  — AED or cardiac monitor
	  — Pulse oximeter
	  — Blood glucometer
	  — Portable suction unit
	  — Automatic stretcher battery (if used)

Communication Devices (each crew member may have a portable radio and/or a direct-connect cell phone)	• All battery-run radios and phones are in working order; all rechargeable radios and phones are fully charged • Radio channels are in working order and radio communications are able to be heard in both directions • If using ePCR equipment, log-in works and software can be accessed with a Wi-Fi or hardwire connection • If using paper charts, stock is available

(Continued)

Table 9.1 *Truck Check Components (Continued)*

Area to Check	Components

Crew Roles & Responsibilities	• Within your crew, be clear about duties and responsibilities so that the execution of your next call will be flawless
	• Share issues that you feel need addressing; trust is essential in a successful EMT team so that in the field you can focus on the challenge at hand
	  — Partners don't always get along, and that can impede ideal patient care. Try to iron out any problems and advise management if necessary.
	  — If you are unsure about how to do a certain procedure, be honest about it, especially if working with an ALS partner. Do not just try to "wing it," as that isn't safe. Ask your partner for direction or explain that you cannot complete the task. Wait until after the call has completed to learn the task; most senior or experienced providers will not mind teaching.
	  — You will be spending long hours with your partner. Everyone has personal preferences about what time to eat, how to prepare the chart, and even critical thinking on patient care. Smooth out these issues beforehand so they are "non-issues" on your calls.
	  — Your partners are your TEAM. Emotions will run high at times, but what matters most is patient care. Collaborate with your partners to give the best possible care.

Once your truck and equipment check are done, be sure to notify the dispatch center with the names of the personnel on board for the shift. This will alert dispatch that you are ready and available to start taking calls.

From Dispatch to Arrival on Scene

After a call is received by the dispatcher, the responding unit is notified (*how* the unit is notified depends on the individual service: loudspeaker, radio, direct-connect cell phone, or in person if the dispatch center and the unit are at the same location). The dispatcher will relay the following information to the responding EMS unit:

- Location of the call
- Nature of the illness or injury
- Special information that may be useful to the responders

The name of the caller and a callback number are not normally broadcast to the responding unit, although the dispatcher does take that information.

En Route to the Scene

When a call is received by EMS from the dispatcher, the following steps take place:

- Crew acknowledges the call, repeating back the location and nature of the emergency; clarification is provided if needed
- Crew then responds quickly and enters vehicle; all personnel secure themselves with seat belts as the driver starts the engine
- Before beginning to move, the driver checks that all doors are closed and all personnel are ready to go

Professional emergency vehicle drivers are physically and mentally fit at all times and alert to their surroundings and circumstances.

Not all EMTs are vehicle drivers. **Emergency vehicle operation** is a separate course from your EMT-Basic education, with special certification. However, certification is often a condition of employment. Additionally, some services will not employ EMTs until they are age 21, due to driving liability rules.

In addition to understanding how to properly operate an emergency vehicle, the driver is also responsible for the following:

- Be intimately familiar with the vehicle you are driving, especially with its particular quirks
- Anticipate the unexpected
- Avoid danger on the road at all costs, i.e., do not let the rush of adrenaline or excited radio traffic overcome your common sense and duty to drive safely
- Tolerate other drivers on the road who may not yield the right of way, in spite of the EMS lights and sirens

All states give certain privileges to emergency vehicles, such as being allowed to drive over the speed limit to a certain extent; however, there are some obvious limitations (with risk of penalty). The general idea is that emergency vehicles must drive with **due regard** for the safety of others. They must:

- Provide adequate warning to others by using the warning devices
- Control the speed of the vehicle to allow other motorists time to react to your warning
- Use emergency lights and sirens judiciously and only as stated in your state protocols
- Use extreme caution for cross traffic when approaching any intersection, regardless of the traffic control. (Some drivers actually push through a red stoplight into the path of an oncoming ambulance, thinking the ambulance is behind them.)

- Be aware that other emergency vehicles may be operating in priority mode at the same time you are and attempting to assert their right of way
- Park the ambulance in a normal manner and not on the sidewalk (unless necessary) or in the fire lane
- Always stop for a school bus with its red lights activated; emergency vehicles never have the right of way in those situations
- Use a police escort only if your EMS team is unfamiliar with the location of the receiving facility, and even then GPS should suffice. Vehicles often inadvertently block the path of the ambulance traveling behind a police escort, so use an escort very sparingly.

In the event of an accident, the driver—not the senior EMT—is responsible for the operation of the vehicle and is personally liable in the event of an accident.

Arrival on Scene

Once the unit is on scene, notify the dispatcher of this fact and give an update if the information you received was incorrect or incomplete. If the number of patients exceeds the capacity of the unit to handle, additional units must be requested at this time and MCI (mass casualty incident) procedures must be initiated.

The driver must position the vehicle safely and far enough away if the scene is hazardous or could become so.

- Crew should scan the scene for safety issues before committing the crew to a course of action, e.g., weapons, lack of police, electrical hazards, hazardous materials, and collapse dangers.
- Once the scene is determined to be safe, approach and assess the patient. If there is a potential hazard, e.g., a vehicle on fire, then move the patient first to safety before doing the assessment. Attempt an appropriate level of cervical spine stabilization, but do not hinder the patient's prompt removal from the unsafe scene.
- Once the patient is safely away from the hazard, begin assessment based on whether it is a trauma or medical scenario and initiate proper treatment.
- When the patient is properly triaged and treated, the next step is transport to an appropriate facility (unless that was earlier determined to be a load-and-go injury and you are already en route).

Moving and Lifting Patients

Identifying and treating patients is always seen as the main goal of prehospital emergency medicine. However, extricating patients from the circumstance that you find them in and transporting them to an appropriate medical facility is often where the real art of this type of medical practice is demonstrated.

When lifting a patient, always do so safely. This requires exact communication with all of those involved. Before attempting to lift a patient, be sure you and your partners have a plan as to how this will be accomplished. For example, if you are moving a patient from a hospital bed to a stretcher, it is often easier to accomplish this by sliding the patient on the sheets of the bed right onto your stretcher. If there are multiple sheets beneath the patient, be sure that you all know whether you are taking all of them or just the top one. It is critical when lifting a patient secured to a backboard or even in raising the stretcher from its lowered position to the transport position that the lifting be done in a coordinated manner. Failure to do so may tip the patient right off the stretcher and complicate his or her injuries.

When lifting a patient from a low to a high position, either on a board or on a stretcher, always use your legs to lift, not your back. This necessitates squatting to a kneeling position and keeping the weight close to your body. Your feet should be far enough apart to give you good balance in both squatting and standing positions. You should grip the stretcher, backboard, or sheets with both hands, using the entire hands and not just the fingers.

The EMT must know her own limitations. If the patient weighs more than can safely be handled by the crew on the scene, additional help must be summoned. Remember, all patient transfers must be done with the safety of the crew and patient as a primary consideration.

Transferring Patients

There are three types of patient transfer, each of which can be subdivided into trauma and non-trauma.

Emergency Transfer

An emergency transfer occurs when speed is the primary consideration because the patient and rescuer are in immediate danger.

- The most common example of this is when a motor vehicle has been involved in an accident, the driver is behind the wheel and unconscious, and the vehicle is on fire. The usual precautions for cervical spine stabilization are secondary to removing the patient from the immediate danger.
- This type of extrication is accomplished by whatever method removes the patient from the danger as quickly as possible. If the patient is not entrapped, grabbing the patient beneath the arms and pulling headfirst, trying to cradle the head and neck against your torso as you do so, is the best method.

Urgent Transfer

An urgent transfer occurs when the situation is unstable but not critical.

- In the same scenario as above, but with only smoke issuing from the engine compartment and no fire visible, you may have time to take some precautions to minimize spinal injury.
- One EMT should attempt to stabilize by holding the head from the rear, if possible, while the second EMT applies a cervical collar. Then, with coordinated motion, the EMTs should pivot the patient so that he may be pulled from the vehicle by the long

axis of the body onto a spine board, which can be placed right on the seat of the vehicle (if possible) to minimize patient motion.

- Once the patient is on the spine board, the patient can be moved away from the vehicle to a safe place as quickly as possible and receive the appropriate treatments.

Nonurgent Transfer

In the nonurgent transfer, when there is no discernible danger, the patient would be stabilized in a Kendrick™ Extrication Device (KED) or a similar type of stabilization device prior to being extricated.

There are two basic types of equipment available for patient transfer.

The main piece of equipment used to effect transfers and lifting is the **main ambulance stretcher**, which has an adjustable height. This stretcher comes in three configurations:

- The one-person-loading stretcher allows one person to place the stretcher from its uppermost position into the ambulance, as the wheeled undercarriage folds in by itself.
- The one-and-a-half-person-loading stretcher has a wheel assembly at the head of the stretcher so that once it is engaged inside the truck, it enables one person to lift the stretcher and patient. The second person only has to lift the undercarriage to its resting position beneath the stretcher.
- The two-person-stretcher requires two EMTs to stand on either side and lower it down into position. Two EMTs then lift it into the truck and together roll it into place.

When a full-size ambulance stretcher cannot be brought to the patient, a **folding stretcher (stair chair)** is used. The patient is secured in a sitting position and then transported to a place where transfer can be made to a main stretcher.

If the patient cannot be placed in a sitting position (e.g., a back or neck injury), they must be secured to a backboard and then transported to the main stretcher.

Once the patient has been loaded into the ambulance, the crew should notify dispatch that they are en route to the receiving facility.

Air Transfer

Local protocols will often dictate when air transport is indicated and how it is to be used. The decision may be made by the incident commander or by the applicable medical control. The driving factors will be the trauma score of the patient and the projected transport time via land vehicle.

Unfortunately, in the real world, many other factors affect the handling of the emergency. Helicopters will not fly in a snowstorm (when EMS calls are frequent and often serious), and helicopters are not always available when they had been expected to be. The crew must make a decision based upon all of these considerations.

If air transfer does happen, the crew must establish a safe landing zone for the helicopter, using the following criteria:

- Must be at least 100 × 100 feet, fairly level, and paved/grass-covered if possible
- Must be able to accommodate a nearby fire truck (required for landing)
- Must be free from overhead obstructions, particularly electrical wires
- Must have emergency lighting if at night and unlit

There are many hazards surrounding the use of a helicopter. If possible, the best practice is to have a designated helicopter landing zone, along with live trainings to prepare for the real-world events.

When working with helicopters, always follow certain safety rules:

- Never approach a helicopter until instructed to do so by the pilot or a helicopter crew member.
- Always approach a helicopter from the front or side in view of the pilot, keeping your head down. Do not approach from the rear (unless that is how it is set up).
- If the helicopter is on a slight slope, be aware that the clearance of the main rotors will be dangerously low on the uphill side and may be unapproachable there.
- Follow the instructions of the pilot/crew members carefully. Since helicopter engines are often left running to save time, the blades are often rotating as the patient is loaded/unloaded. It is imperative that you do exactly as the crew requests.

The last step is reporting: you (EMT) and your crew should notify the incoming flight team of the patient's status and specific needs. This will allow them time to determine which equipment they wish to offload from the aircraft and bring to the patient versus what to leave on board.

Once the patient has been loaded, following the flight crew instructions the ambulance crew is now free to end their portion of the call and begin the charting and decontamination process. This is one of the instances in which the ambulance crew often does not do a final handover to hospital personnel, as they have now transferred the patient care to a higher level of care and provider. At this point, once the ambulance has been restocked and cleaned they may notify dispatch that they are available for another emergency call.

En Route to the Receiving Facility

Once en route to the receiving facility, the driver notifies dispatch of that fact, and the EMT responsible for treating the patient collects the information necessary to notify the receiving facility. It is important to paint as clear a picture as possible so that the receiving facility knows the condition of the patient en route and can prepare accordingly. Additionally, while en route, do the following:

- Comfort the patient and provide assurance that optimal care is being given. A patient will quickly sense if you are unsure of yourself, so be confident in your communication.
- Continue to monitor vital signs throughout the trip.

Communication Basics

Providing emergency medical services is a joint effort involving many people, and the success of an endeavor is predicated upon clear and precise communications between the elements of the EMS system.

- EMS calls usually begin with a phone call to an emergency dispatcher. This call may be to a dedicated emergency line, a 911 call center, or even a routine phone line.
- The dispatcher is responsible for accurately taking down the location and nature of the call and, if qualified, giving pre-arrival instructions.
- This information may be relayed to a second dispatcher who actually dispatches the nearest appropriate EMS unit, usually by two-way radio, and who is responsible for transmitting the information received by the call taker.
- The EMS unit will give updates and changes in status back to the dispatcher, such as "en route," "arrive on scene," etc.

Communications Technology

The EMT is also responsible for notifying the receiving hospital of patient information and in many cases for seeking guidance from a physician as to performing procedures described in the applicable protocols.

Historically this task was done by two-way radio but is now often done by cell phone.

Clear communication between all personnel involved in the EMS system is paramount. This is accomplished through the following:

- Communications equipment should be checked at the beginning of each shift to ensure its proper functioning.
- Backup systems (and redundant systems) are needed so that all elements of public safety can communicate with each other as needed, even in the event of a large-scale disaster.
- When communicating via radio, know exactly what it is you want to communicate before starting to speak.
  - Speak slowly and clearly, using proper terminology.
  - When listening to/receiving information, remember to release the push-to-talk (PTT) switch.
  - If your system is using radio repeaters to allow for long range communication, you may have to wait a few seconds before transmitting, which also delays the reception of incoming radio traffic.

There are different types of radio systems that EMS utilizes to transmit information to each other or receiving hospitals.

- *Simplex* transmits and receives messages on the same frequency.
- *Duplex* transmits and receives messages on different frequencies, which is referred to as a channel.

- *Multiplex* has the capability to transmit two signals at the same time. An example would be when a paramedic can both talk to the physician and transmit an EKG at the same time.

- *Repeater* receives a signal and retransmits it. They are used to extend transmissions so that the signal can cover longer distances or be received on the other side of an obstruction such as a mountain or valley. This is how units may stay in contact with their base station from many miles away and still be heard clearly.

With two-way radio, various EMS units may share a common frequency. In those cases, be mindful of radio courtesy; if someone transmits while another unit is already transmitting, both conversations may become unintelligible.

Research has shown that a **lack of communication between public safety units** is highly problematic and significant during major disasters. EMS systems must take these issues into account when designing and utilizing communications systems.

Communication and Confidentiality

When communicating over public safety radio, be sure to maintain patient confidentiality. Radio frequencies are open to (and often monitored by) the general public and news media, so be sure not to reveal a patient's name or other identifying information. Keep all information neutral.

A good idea of information to include in a radio report without compromising confidentiality includes:

- Age and gender of patient
- Chief complaint
- Last or most relevant set of vital signs recorded
- Treatment given or in progress with the patient's response to it
- Any orders, such as asking to administer certain medications, from medical control
- Medical history or medications pertinent to the situation
- Estimated time of arrival (ETA) to facility if transporting

As you become more experienced and confident in your radio reporting style, you will come up with a basic setup of a radio report that will address all the bullet points above and last approximately 2–3 minutes or less. A sample radio report could sound as follows:

"This is EMS unit 27 en route to your hospital with a 5 minutes ETA. I am transporting a 67-year-old male BLS, alert and oriented ×4, who is complaining of a hand laceration due to a fall from a stepladder with no loss of consciousness. He is not currently on any blood thinners. His last set of vitals are BP 132/76 mm Hg, respiratory rate of 18, pulse rate of 86, SpO2 of 100% on room air. Bleeding is controlled by pressure and bandages. Do you require anything further? See you in 5 minutes."

When you arrive at the receiving facility, the triage nurse may or may not have received your report, so you will tell him in person what you have told the person on the radio and then follow the nurse's directions to transfer your patient to the emergency department's care.

Radio Codes

Radio codes are specific words or numbers assigned to each medical issue or injury a patient could be experiencing. It is a way to protect confidentiality over the radio frequencies in case other people are listening in. Confidential information should be passed by more secure transmissions, such as cell phones.

Radio codes vary from location to location, and even from service to service. Dispatch systems, which use confidential codes for sensitive calls, e.g., attempted suicide or sexual assault, should make sure that all trainees are well-versed in the codes and how they are used. For example, a service may dispatch your unit as follows:

- You are dispatched to a code 19, which could mean respiratory distress.
- You would then respond code 7, which means "en route with lights and sirens."
- When you get on scene, you would radio dispatch and say you are code 10, meaning "you have arrived."
- When you transport the patient, you would say that you are code 20, meaning "en route to the hospital."

As you can see, this can be very confusing and time-consuming, especially if the EMT is not completely familiar and comfortable with the meaning of each code.
If you are working for a company that still uses radio codes, it is up to the EMT to be familiar with and know how to use them properly.

One service may use a completely different set of radio codes than another service less than 10 miles away. Therefore, the National Incident Management System (NIMS) prohibits the use of radio codes during a multiple-agency operation. During an event that involves more than one agency, personnel are required to use "plain English," which allows all communication to be easily understood. Since this policy (law) has been implemented, many EMS services are starting to adopt this policy as their standard.

Patient Drop-Off and Post-Run

During transport, while patient care is being performed, the EMT must also be thinking about what to communicate in the prehospital radio report (before arrival at the receiving facility) and in the hospital bedside handover report (upon arrival).

The **prehospital radio report** (done orally via radio or cell phone; not written) provides the following:

- A brief rundown of how long the hospital has before the ambulance will arrive
- Age and gender of the patient
- Description of the medical or trauma problem the patient is experiencing
- Treatment the patient was given (by EMTs) upon arrival at the scene and response to it
- Additional resources that may be required at the hospital, i.e., security for a combative behavioral patient or additional personnel to help with CPR if the patient is in cardiac arrest

Patient Drop-Off

Once at the receiving facility, the driver notifies dispatch of their arrival and goes to the rear of the vehicle to assist in removing the patient. The patient is brought to the triage area and transferred to hospital care by the direction of the receiving nurse or physician. A **complete oral report** (or **bedside handover report** [or just bedside report]) is given to the initial hospital caregiver, along with a copy of the PCR (written or electronic format) containing the pertinent information from the assessments, vital signs, and EMT interventions.

Patient care is then transferred to the hospital staff, and once the EMT has confirmed that the hospital staff have all the information they need only then is prehospital care terminated. The EMT may then move onto the cleaning and resupplying of the ambulance.

Remember that unless the EMT has given a report and gained confirmation that hospital personnel (of an equal or higher level of certification) will continue care of the patient, the EMS provider may not leave their patient. This is considered abandonment and poor provider judgement. EMS providers must assure that there is another medical provider that steps in and continues care for their patients, not just leave them on a hospital bed and hope someone comes along or checks on them. Legally speaking, there could also be prosecution for this act if charges were pressed by the patient or hospital.

Post-Run

Once you are clear of the call, do the following:

- Restock the truck if that wasn't already done at the hospital
- Complete the run report after obtaining the times from the dispatcher
- File the run report according to local protocols regarding confidentiality of patient-care information
- Restock disposable supplies
- Clean linens that are used for the stretcher

Once everything has been cleaned, disinfected, and restocked, the unit is available for another run. The last step is to notify dispatch that the unit is back in service.

Special Situations

Weapons of Mass Destruction

It is a sad truth in the post-9/11 world that EMS providers will be on the front line of a terrorist attack involving weapons of mass destruction. These weapons fall into five categories and are remembered by the acronym *CBRNE* (*"SeeBurn-E"*):

- **C**hemical
- **B**iological
- **R**adiological
- **N**uclear
- **E**xplosives

The primary concern of the responding EMS personnel should be for their own safety. Dangers from these types of attacks are not always apparent, however, so EMS personnel must always be on high guard.

Table 9.2 *CBRNE Categories*

Category	Components
Chemical	- Blistering agents (mustard gas, lewisite) - Nerve agents (sarin, tabun) - Blood agents (cyanogen chloride, hydrogen cyanide) - Choking agents (phosgene, chlorine)
Biological	- Anthrax - Tularemia - Smallpox - Ricin - Other bacterial and viral agents
Radioactive	- Explosive device that releases radioactive isotopes to pollute an area with radiation - Dispersed by so-called "dirty bomb"
Nuclear	- Major explosive device with resultant radiologic contamination; profoundly devastating - Explosion is created by changing atoms (either split or fused to create new atoms), which causes extremely significant destruction within seconds or minutes
Explosive	- Bombs: regular, pipe, pressure cooker - Improvised explosive devices (IED) - Anything that can burst apart and cause widespread damage with intent to harm

These types of attacks require intervention of specifically trained personnel that falls beyond the scope of this exam. However, all public safety personnel must be aware of these types of weapons and be prepared to provide backup support as needed in the event of a terrorist event.

Mass Casualty Incidents

Any incident that involves more patients than a single unit can handle is considered to be a mass casualty incident (MCI). This can be as few as 2–3 people or as many as 100+.

After determining that the scene is safe, whoever was on scene first must analyze the number and severity of injured patients.

Doing Triage

Triage identifies the most severely injured patients with the greatest chance of surviving. It helps to sort a large number of people in an unemotional way into categories during what is likely to be a very emotional and chaotic event.

Triage can be difficult because minimal treatment is provided throughout the process, which can be very counterintuitive for EMS providers who by their very nature want to help as many people as possible. In an MCI, the greatest good needs to be offered to the greatest number of people.

This ideology works efficiently to separate patients into various categories quickly, but can be quite emotionally traumatic for those doing triage, especially if dealing with children. Acknowledging this part of the job is half of the mental battle, but is important to know. It is one thing to learn about the system but it is quite a different thing to do it in real life, where you may have the very real job of declaring a patient deceased, even if they are taking shallow breaths.

The crew on scene is often referred to as "command." They will be in charge of getting the triage process started and also directing incoming units where to stage or how to approach the scene. Once more assistance is on scene, dedicated treatment and sorting areas should be identified and set up so that patients can start flowing through.

There are a few methods of triage, and each service uses a different one. However, the most common methods include:

- **START**: Simple Triage and Rapid Treatment
- **JumpSTART**: pediatric-specific level of START triage
- **SALT**: Sort, Assess, Lifesaving interventions, Treatment/Transport

Regardless of the system used, patients are identified by a color system. This can be achieved by commercially made triage tags, colored tape, or other means. The most commonly used colors are:

- **Red**: require immediate transport
- **Yellow**: urgent, but transport can be delayed
- **Green**: non-life-threatening injuries; "walking wounded"
- **Black/gray**: deceased or injuries that are too extensive
- **White**: no injuries

Awaiting Transport

Once patients have been triaged, the patients need a place to await transport. During this time, some initial treatment may be started if there are resources available.

- On smaller scenes, the arriving ambulance crews might be directed to a specific area to find their patient.
- With larger events, a treatment area and loading area should be identified and constructed. This can be accomplished with tents, colored tarps, or chalked-off areas.

Finally, consider where the patients should be transported. An MCI can overwhelm local hospitals, especially smaller ones. Notify nearby hospitals immediately, i.e., as soon as an event has been identified; that will give them time to prepare for multiple patients at once. Keep in mind the following questions:

- How many patients require transport?
- How many hospitals are available to receive these patients, and what is each hospital's capability, i.e., is it a trauma center? Community hospital? Pediatric-specific?
- How many EMS units are available to assist with the transports?

Practice Set

1. Ambulances should be supplied with

    A. only those supplies that the service can afford.

    B. all the supplies necessary for the operations for which the ambulance is licensed.

    C. an emergency childbirth kit.

    D. safety equipment mandated by the licensing authority.

2. Due regard is best described as

    A. forcing people to pull over for you when using lights and sirens.

    B. following local traffic rules, even during an emergency.

    C. making sure your ambulance is in working order.

    D. slowing down at stop signs, then proceeding through the intersection.

3. As you begin your shift, you receive an emergency dispatch for a patient in respiratory distress at a local nursing home. You have not yet performed the mandatory truck check. What should you do?

    A. Disregard the check and let the next shift do it

    B. Do not respond to any calls until the check is completed

    C. Respond to the call and perform the check when you return in service

    D. Have the driver perform the check while you assess the patient

4. Which of the following does NOT rely on an electrical battery?

    A. Pulse oximeter

    B. Portable oxygen tank

    C. Glucometer

    D. Portable suction unit

5. Your EMS radio announces, "Rescue 1, respond to 123 Main Street for a man fallen off a ladder with head laceration, possibly unconscious, time out 15:30 hours." Your response to dispatch should be

    A. "10-4."

    B. "Roger."

    C. "Rescue 1 responding emergently to 123 Main Street for a male possibly unconscious with a head laceration."

    D. "Rescue 1 responding with two EMTs, basic life support only, lights and sirens, to 123 Main Street in Anytown for a male who has fallen off of a ladder and has a possible skull fracture. We are responding at 15:31 hours. Do you copy, dispatch?"

6. The yellow triage tag color most commonly means the patient

    A. is soon to be deceased without treatment.

    B. has a serious injury but can wait to be transported by another responding unit.

    C. needs to have additional airway maneuvers done.

    D. needs to be transported immediately.

7. You respond emergently to a motor vehicle accident. Arriving on scene, you notice that a car has struck a fuel tank truck broadside, and liquid is running downhill toward you. The best place to park your ambulance is

   A. at the spot you first noticed the liquid.
   B. past the vehicle, uphill from the liquid spill.
   C. directly next to the vehicle to expedite patient care and transfer.
   D. 250 feet from the crash.

8. When should you notify the receiving facility of a critically ill patient?

   A. At the time of dispatch
   B. En route to the hospital
   C. Never
   D. At the conclusion of the rapid assessment

Answers and Explanations

1. B

The minimum list of supplies is usually mandated by the licensing authority, but the service should be carrying everything necessary for the operations for which the ambulance is licensed, whether basic life support, advanced life support, pediatric transport, neonate transport, etc. (C) and (D) are partially correct since any BLS ambulance should have them, but (B) is the best answer.

2. B

Regardless of whether lights or sirens are being used, an emergency vehicle operator must always follow local traffic rules and posted speed limits, which makes (B) the answer. Certain allowances may be afforded to EMS by local police, such as allowances over the speed limit within reason, but it is not always a guarantee and it is up to the driver to exercise caution in all operations of the vehicle. (C) is part of the shift truck check. (A) and (D) are dangerous maneuvers that should not be completed.

3. B

Despite the seriousness of a dispatch, no calls should be run without confirming that all equipment is present, accounted for, and in working order. If a crew is missing full oxygen cylinders or other oxygen adjuncts, they will be of no use to a patient in respiratory distress. (C) is a tempting answer given the dispatch but not the most correct answer in this scenario. A call for respiratory distress is going to require both crew members, so (D) is also incorrect. Never do (A), as you are responsible for your shift and making sure that everything is there.

4. B

The portable oxygen tank does not rely on an electric battery. (A) and (C) are definitely battery operated. (D) is questionable, since portable suction units can be either electrically or manually operated. Again, all answers must be read and the best answer chosen.

5. C

If the information was not heard properly, the unit could respond to the wrong location, so repeating the dispatch information is always prudent. (A) and (B) are merely acknowledgments. (D) is too long, relays back information that is not pertinent, and attempts a diagnosis without even seeing the patient. This ties up the radio frequency unnecessarily.

6. B

The correct answer is (B), with a delay in transport. The patient may have serious injuries but is stable enough to be transported later by an additional unit.

7. B

The uphill parking place will put your vehicle out of the path of this potentially dangerous spill. (A) is incorrect because the liquid is continuing to spill and will soon be underneath your vehicle, putting it directly in a hazardous situation. (C) is incorrect since parking that close to a leaking fuel truck is dangerous to the vehicle, crew, and patient. (D) is incomplete and should be discarded.

8. B

En route to the receiving facility is the correct answer. (A) is incorrect, since at the time of dispatch you do not have enough information. (D) is incorrect, since after the rapid assessment you still do not have all of the required information.

Full-Length Practice Test and Explanations

Answer Sheet

Remove (or photocopy) this answer sheet and use it to complete the practice test.
See the answer key following the test when finished. For an analysis of your score,
see "Your Practice Test Score," following the answer explanation section.

1. Ⓐ Ⓑ Ⓒ Ⓓ	31. Ⓐ Ⓑ Ⓒ Ⓓ	61. Ⓐ Ⓑ Ⓒ Ⓓ	91. Ⓐ Ⓑ Ⓒ Ⓓ	121. Ⓐ Ⓑ Ⓒ Ⓓ
2. Ⓐ Ⓑ Ⓒ Ⓓ	32. Ⓐ Ⓑ Ⓒ Ⓓ	62. Ⓐ Ⓑ Ⓒ Ⓓ	92. Ⓐ Ⓑ Ⓒ Ⓓ	122. Ⓐ Ⓑ Ⓒ Ⓓ
3. Ⓐ Ⓑ Ⓒ Ⓓ	33. Ⓐ Ⓑ Ⓒ Ⓓ	63. Ⓐ Ⓑ Ⓒ Ⓓ	93. Ⓐ Ⓑ Ⓒ Ⓓ	123. Ⓐ Ⓑ Ⓒ Ⓓ
4. Ⓐ Ⓑ Ⓒ Ⓓ	34. Ⓐ Ⓑ Ⓒ Ⓓ	64. Ⓐ Ⓑ Ⓒ Ⓓ	94. Ⓐ Ⓑ Ⓒ Ⓓ	124. Ⓐ Ⓑ Ⓒ Ⓓ
5. Ⓐ Ⓑ Ⓒ Ⓓ	35. Ⓐ Ⓑ Ⓒ Ⓓ	65. Ⓐ Ⓑ Ⓒ Ⓓ	95. Ⓐ Ⓑ Ⓒ Ⓓ	125. Ⓐ Ⓑ Ⓒ Ⓓ
6. Ⓐ Ⓑ Ⓒ Ⓓ	36. Ⓐ Ⓑ Ⓒ Ⓓ	66. Ⓐ Ⓑ Ⓒ Ⓓ	96. Ⓐ Ⓑ Ⓒ Ⓓ	126. Ⓐ Ⓑ Ⓒ Ⓓ
7. Ⓐ Ⓑ Ⓒ Ⓓ	37. Ⓐ Ⓑ Ⓒ Ⓓ	67. Ⓐ Ⓑ Ⓒ Ⓓ	97. Ⓐ Ⓑ Ⓒ Ⓓ	127. Ⓐ Ⓑ Ⓒ Ⓓ
8. Ⓐ Ⓑ Ⓒ Ⓓ	38. Ⓐ Ⓑ Ⓒ Ⓓ	68. Ⓐ Ⓑ Ⓒ Ⓓ	98. Ⓐ Ⓑ Ⓒ Ⓓ	128. Ⓐ Ⓑ Ⓒ Ⓓ
9. Ⓐ Ⓑ Ⓒ Ⓓ	39. Ⓐ Ⓑ Ⓒ Ⓓ	69. Ⓐ Ⓑ Ⓒ Ⓓ	99. Ⓐ Ⓑ Ⓒ Ⓓ	129. Ⓐ Ⓑ Ⓒ Ⓓ
10. Ⓐ Ⓑ Ⓒ Ⓓ	40. Ⓐ Ⓑ Ⓒ Ⓓ	70. Ⓐ Ⓑ Ⓒ Ⓓ	100. Ⓐ Ⓑ Ⓒ Ⓓ	130. Ⓐ Ⓑ Ⓒ Ⓓ
11. Ⓐ Ⓑ Ⓒ Ⓓ	41. Ⓐ Ⓑ Ⓒ Ⓓ	71. Ⓐ Ⓑ Ⓒ Ⓓ	101. Ⓐ Ⓑ Ⓒ Ⓓ	131. Ⓐ Ⓑ Ⓒ Ⓓ
12. Ⓐ Ⓑ Ⓒ Ⓓ	42. Ⓐ Ⓑ Ⓒ Ⓓ	72. Ⓐ Ⓑ Ⓒ Ⓓ	102. Ⓐ Ⓑ Ⓒ Ⓓ	132. Ⓐ Ⓑ Ⓒ Ⓓ
13. Ⓐ Ⓑ Ⓒ Ⓓ	43. Ⓐ Ⓑ Ⓒ Ⓓ	73. Ⓐ Ⓑ Ⓒ Ⓓ	103. Ⓐ Ⓑ Ⓒ Ⓓ	133. Ⓐ Ⓑ Ⓒ Ⓓ
14. Ⓐ Ⓑ Ⓒ Ⓓ	44. Ⓐ Ⓑ Ⓒ Ⓓ	74. Ⓐ Ⓑ Ⓒ Ⓓ	104. Ⓐ Ⓑ Ⓒ Ⓓ	134. Ⓐ Ⓑ Ⓒ Ⓓ
15. Ⓐ Ⓑ Ⓒ Ⓓ	45. Ⓐ Ⓑ Ⓒ Ⓓ	75. Ⓐ Ⓑ Ⓒ Ⓓ	105. Ⓐ Ⓑ Ⓒ Ⓓ	135. Ⓐ Ⓑ Ⓒ Ⓓ
16. Ⓐ Ⓑ Ⓒ Ⓓ	46. Ⓐ Ⓑ Ⓒ Ⓓ	76. Ⓐ Ⓑ Ⓒ Ⓓ	106. Ⓐ Ⓑ Ⓒ Ⓓ	136. Ⓐ Ⓑ Ⓒ Ⓓ
17. Ⓐ Ⓑ Ⓒ Ⓓ	47. Ⓐ Ⓑ Ⓒ Ⓓ	77. Ⓐ Ⓑ Ⓒ Ⓓ	107. Ⓐ Ⓑ Ⓒ Ⓓ	137. Ⓐ Ⓑ Ⓒ Ⓓ
18. Ⓐ Ⓑ Ⓒ Ⓓ	48. Ⓐ Ⓑ Ⓒ Ⓓ	78. Ⓐ Ⓑ Ⓒ Ⓓ	108. Ⓐ Ⓑ Ⓒ Ⓓ	138. Ⓐ Ⓑ Ⓒ Ⓓ
19. Ⓐ Ⓑ Ⓒ Ⓓ	49. Ⓐ Ⓑ Ⓒ Ⓓ	79. Ⓐ Ⓑ Ⓒ Ⓓ	109. Ⓐ Ⓑ Ⓒ Ⓓ	139. Ⓐ Ⓑ Ⓒ Ⓓ
20. Ⓐ Ⓑ Ⓒ Ⓓ	50. Ⓐ Ⓑ Ⓒ Ⓓ	80. Ⓐ Ⓑ Ⓒ Ⓓ	110. Ⓐ Ⓑ Ⓒ Ⓓ	140. Ⓐ Ⓑ Ⓒ Ⓓ
21. Ⓐ Ⓑ Ⓒ Ⓓ	51. Ⓐ Ⓑ Ⓒ Ⓓ	81. Ⓐ Ⓑ Ⓒ Ⓓ	111. Ⓐ Ⓑ Ⓒ Ⓓ	141. Ⓐ Ⓑ Ⓒ Ⓓ
22. Ⓐ Ⓑ Ⓒ Ⓓ	52. Ⓐ Ⓑ Ⓒ Ⓓ	82. Ⓐ Ⓑ Ⓒ Ⓓ	112. Ⓐ Ⓑ Ⓒ Ⓓ	142. Ⓐ Ⓑ Ⓒ Ⓓ
23. Ⓐ Ⓑ Ⓒ Ⓓ	53. Ⓐ Ⓑ Ⓒ Ⓓ	83. Ⓐ Ⓑ Ⓒ Ⓓ	113. Ⓐ Ⓑ Ⓒ Ⓓ	143. Ⓐ Ⓑ Ⓒ Ⓓ
24. Ⓐ Ⓑ Ⓒ Ⓓ	54. Ⓐ Ⓑ Ⓒ Ⓓ	84. Ⓐ Ⓑ Ⓒ Ⓓ	114. Ⓐ Ⓑ Ⓒ Ⓓ	144. Ⓐ Ⓑ Ⓒ Ⓓ
25. Ⓐ Ⓑ Ⓒ Ⓓ	55. Ⓐ Ⓑ Ⓒ Ⓓ	85. Ⓐ Ⓑ Ⓒ Ⓓ	115. Ⓐ Ⓑ Ⓒ Ⓓ	145. Ⓐ Ⓑ Ⓒ Ⓓ
26. Ⓐ Ⓑ Ⓒ Ⓓ	56. Ⓐ Ⓑ Ⓒ Ⓓ	86. Ⓐ Ⓑ Ⓒ Ⓓ	116. Ⓐ Ⓑ Ⓒ Ⓓ	146. Ⓐ Ⓑ Ⓒ Ⓓ
27. Ⓐ Ⓑ Ⓒ Ⓓ	57. Ⓐ Ⓑ Ⓒ Ⓓ	87. Ⓐ Ⓑ Ⓒ Ⓓ	117. Ⓐ Ⓑ Ⓒ Ⓓ	147. Ⓐ Ⓑ Ⓒ Ⓓ
28. Ⓐ Ⓑ Ⓒ Ⓓ	58. Ⓐ Ⓑ Ⓒ Ⓓ	88. Ⓐ Ⓑ Ⓒ Ⓓ	118. Ⓐ Ⓑ Ⓒ Ⓓ	148. Ⓐ Ⓑ Ⓒ Ⓓ
29. Ⓐ Ⓑ Ⓒ Ⓓ	59. Ⓐ Ⓑ Ⓒ Ⓓ	89. Ⓐ Ⓑ Ⓒ Ⓓ	119. Ⓐ Ⓑ Ⓒ Ⓓ	149. Ⓐ Ⓑ Ⓒ Ⓓ
30. Ⓐ Ⓑ Ⓒ Ⓓ	60. Ⓐ Ⓑ Ⓒ Ⓓ	90. Ⓐ Ⓑ Ⓒ Ⓓ	120. Ⓐ Ⓑ Ⓒ Ⓓ	150. Ⓐ Ⓑ Ⓒ Ⓓ

PRACTICE
TEST

Practice Test

1. Which of the following is an example of an unsafe scene for an EMT to enter?

   A. 54-year-old male with difficulty breathing

   B. 23-year-old female with abdominal pain

   C. 18-year-old male with a gunshot wound to the chest

   D. 4-year-old male with leg pain

2. The arterioles connect the _____ and the capillaries.

   A. veins

   B. venules

   C. arteries

   D. vena cavae

3. Which of the following patients is at greatest risk for hypothermia?

   A. 30-year-old firefighter

   B. 70-year-old librarian

   C. 45-year-old EMT

   D. 11-year-old skier

4. Which of the following is NOT one of the five stages of grief?

   A. Denial

   B. Anger

   C. Crying

   D. Acceptance

5. The zygomatic bones are located in the

   A. chest.

   B. lower leg.

   C. back.

   D. face.

6. Which of the following federal laws was created to prevent "patient dumping" and the practice of denying treatment to patients with no insurance?

   A. Emergency Medical Treatment and Active Labor Act (EMTALA)

   B. The White Paper Act

   C. Health Insurance Portability and Accountability Act (HIPAA)

   D. The Medical Practice Act of 1988

7. When using air transport, the EMT should approach a helicopter

   A. from the uphill side.

   B. from the rear.

   C. only when instructed by a helicopter crew member.

   D. under no circumstances, but instead allow the crew to come to them.

8. Which of the following should be noted as insignificant in conducting the patient assessment?

   A. Medication bottles

   B. Comments of bystanders and family members

   C. Physical condition of the patient

   D. Patient's medical insurance

9. Which of the following is NOT a component of the Glasgow Coma Scale?

   A. Eye opening

   B. Verbal response

   C. Motor response

   D. Grimace response

10. You have an EMT student riding with you today. She is studying for an upcoming test and cannot remember a legal term. She recalls that you must have four elements in order to prove this type of claim. She knows that the four elements are duty, breach of duty, proximate cause, and harm caused. What term is she studying?

    A. Abandonment

    B. Tort

    C. Negligence

    D. Malpractice

11. The head is _____ to the chest.

    A. inferior

    B. anterior

    C. superior

    D. posterior

12. What does the "A" stand for in DCAP-BTLS?

    A. Angulation

    B. Arterial bleeding

    C. Alert response

    D. Abrasions

13. There are _____ vertebrae in the lumbar section.

    A. 5

    B. 7

    C. 12

    D. 14

14. Signs and symptoms of post-traumatic stress disorder (PTSD) include the following EXCEPT:

    A. Loss of sexual desire

    B. Loss of appetite

    C. Loss of interest in work

    D. Loss of spontaneity

15. What does the letter "G" in the APGAR score represent?

    A. Grating

    B. Grimace

    C. Guarding

    D. Gurgling

16. You are dispatched to a motor-vehicle accident on a local city street. You respond emergently and arrive on scene with suitable precautions. The police are also on scene. There is one victim, a female seated in the car. Her car backed into another car as she was pulling out of her driveway at low speed. As you approach, she advises you that she is 36 weeks pregnant with her first child. She says she has no injuries, is not hemorrhaging, and is not in any pain; however, she wishes to be checked out at the hospital. In what position should she be transported?

    A. Trendelenburg

    B. Fowler

    C. Semi-Fowler

    D. Right lateral recumbent

17. You respond to an 18-year-old male who is threatening suicide. The fire department states that before you arrived, the patient told them that he wanted to kill himself. Now, the patient says he does not want to hurt himself but he just wants to be left alone. Which of the following is the most appropriate treatment?

    A. Explain the risks of staying at home with suicidal thoughts, and then have the patient sign a re-fusal form if he appears mentally competent

    B. Inform the patient that because he told the fire department that he wants to hurt himself, he will have to go to the hospital, then have the police department assist you with ensuring that the patient is transported to the hospital

    C. Find out if the patient can make an appointment with his personal doctor, and then confirm that he does have an appointment before you clear the scene and return to the station

    D. Since the patient did not tell you personally that he wants to kill himself, you must allow him to make his own decisions; explain to him that he needs to get mental health assistance

18. You respond to a call for a 20-year-old female acting strangely in a supermarket. You respond nonemergently and are met by the police, who request transport of the patient to a hospital for a psychological evaluation. The patient is ballet dancing in the aisles, bowing, and throwing kisses to an imaginary audience. As you approach, she smiles and introduces you to her imaginary dancing partner, Rudolf Nureyev. What should you do next?

    A. Pretend to shake Mr. Nureyev's hand

    B. Wrap your arms around the patient and force her to the stretcher

    C. Gently explain to her that there is no Mr. Nureyev dancing with her

    D. Tackle the patient and assist the police in hand-cuffing her hands behind her back

19. A neonate will normally have _____ pulse rates and respiratory rates than an infant.

    A. higher

    B. lower

    C. more irregular

    D. less irregular

20. Most EMTs are injured at which of the following types of calls?

    A. Domestic violence calls

    B. Motor vehicle accidents

    C. Industrial accidents

    D. In-station accidents

21. Veins are blood vessels that carry deoxygenated blood _____ the heart.

    A. into

    B. away from

    C. toward

    D. from the lungs to

22. Which of the following is NOT a type of muscle?

    A. Voluntary

    B. Involuntary

    C. Cardiac

    D. Regulatory

23. Which of the following is NOT a component of the SAMPLE history?

    A. Signs and symptoms

    B. Allergies

    C. Medications

    D. Pulse rate

24. When should EMS communication equipment be checked?

    A. Daily

    B. Monthly

    C. Weekly

    D. At the start of every shift

25. The first thing to consider when arriving on scene of an emergency call is

    A. scene safety.

    B. universal precautions.

    C. airway.

    D. breathing.

26. A "bulls-eye" or starring pattern of a windshield that occurred during a motor vehicle crash would indicate that the patient may suffer from what kind of serious injury?

    A. Laceration to the scalp

    B. Broken nose from the impact

    C. Concussion

    D. Cervical and spinal damage

27. Once you have determined that the scene is safe and you are wearing the proper universal precautions, the next thing to be checked is

    A. airway.

    B. breathing.

    C. circulation.

    D. level of consciousness.

28. Which of the following is NOT a level of consciousness?

    A. alert

    B. conscious

    C. active

    D. oriented

29. Perfusion in patient assessment refers to the amount of

    A. fluid in the lungs.

    B. oxygen in the hemoglobin.

    C. urine in the bladder.

    D. blood in the heart.

30. Your patient has a core body temperature of 91°F. This temperature indicates what stage of hypothermia?

    A. Severe

    B. Moderate

    C. Mild

    D. Irreversible

31. You are dispatched to a residence for a man down. You respond emergently and arrive on scene wearing suitable precautions. The scene is safe, and the patient's wife advises you that he is undergoing chemotherapy for lung cancer. The patient presents on the primary assessment as unresponsive reflex. His airway is open, he is breathing spontaneously at a rate of 12, and he has a weak, thready pulse rate of 100. A non-rebreather mask is placed on the patient at a flow rate of 15 lpm. Your transport time to the nearest hospital emergency department is 30 minutes, but there is an ALS unit 15 minutes out. Your next step should be which of the following?

    A. Call for an ALS intercept

    B. Begin priority transport

    C. Administer 0.3 mg epinephrine subcutaneously

    D. Request an air transport

32. The letter "Q" in the acronym OPQRST stands for

    A. quantity.

    B. quality.

    C. quasi.

    D. quick.

33. After the focused trauma assessment is completed on a serious trauma patient, the assessment should be rechecked every

    A. 2 minutes.
    B. 3 minutes.
    C. 5 minutes.
    D. 15 minutes.

34. Which of the following best describes an indirect force injury?

    A. When an object strikes a person and transfers all of its energy to the point of impact
    B. When a force is applied to one region of the body but causes an injury in another region of the body
    C. When a patient has a medical condition that causes weakened bones to fracture
    D. When a penetrating injury leads to a fracture or other musculoskeletal injury

35. In the mnemonic DCAP-BTLS, the letter "B" stands for

    A. bruising.
    B. brittleness.
    C. burns.
    D. broken.

36. A patient viewed from the side is bisected by the

    A. midaxillary line.
    B. midclavicular line.
    C. midsternal line.
    D. horizontal plane.

37. You are dispatched to a man who has fallen from a garage roof. You respond emergently and arrive on scene wearing suitable precautions. The scene is safe. The patient is a 32-year-old male who is conscious but confused as to what events happened as to cause the injury. You are holding stabilization while your partner completes the focused trauma assessment. Which device should be applied following the focused assessment of the head and neck?

    A. Head blocks
    B. Hare traction device
    C. NRB mask
    D. Cervical collar

38. The Good Samaritan Act is a

    A. religious doctrine.
    B. statute that minimizes liability for certain acts.
    C. good deed done by an EMT.
    D. law that protects EMTs 100% of the time from getting sued.

39. While en route to the hospital with a critically ill patient, how often should you repeat vital signs as part of ongoing assessment?

    A. Every 1 minute
    B. Every 3 minutes
    C. Every 5 minutes
    D. Every 10 minutes

40. The "U" in the mnemonic AVPU means

    A. uniform.
    B. unequivocal.
    C. unknown.
    D. unresponsive.

41. Which of the following should never be given over the two-way radio system?

    A. The location of a call

    B. The nature of a call

    C. The patient's name

    D. The EMT's name

42. Which of the following is NOT a required part of a prehospital care report?

    A. Patient's name

    B. Patient's date of birth

    C. Patient's gender

    D. Patient's emergency contact name

43. You are dispatched to the local high school for an eye injury. You respond emergently and arrive on scene, the scene is safe, and you are wearing suitable precautions. You are directed to the nurse's office, where you find a 16-year-old male with a pencil stuck in his left eye. All vital signs are normal, and there is no other injury. You should dress and bandage

    A. his left eye.

    B. both eyes.

    C. his entire upper head.

    D. A dressing is not indicated.

44. Which of the following situations do you NOT have to report to an appropriate state agency if you become aware of it?

    A. Child abuse

    B. Sexual abuse

    C. Elder abuse

    D. Alcohol abuse

45. When is the umbilical cord cut?

    A. Immediately after the baby is delivered

    B. When it ceases pulsing

    C. When the placenta is delivered

    D. At the hospital

46. Which of the following is NOT a sign or symptom of hypovolemic shock?

    A. Hypotension

    B. Excessive thirst

    C. Tachypnea

    D. Hypertension

47. A competent patient may refuse which of the following procedures?

    A. Cervical stabilization with a cervical collar

    B. Spinal immobilization with a spine board

    C. Medication administration

    D. All of the above

48. Which of the following oxygen delivery devices normally provides 24–40% oxygen when attached to supplemental oxygen?

    A. Nasal cannula

    B. Simple face mask

    C. Non-rebreather mask

    D. Bag-valve mask

49. SIDS normally occurs between the ages of

    A. 0 and 1.

    B. 1 and 2.

    C. 2 and 3.

    D. 3 and 4.

50. An impaled object should never be removed unless

    A. ordered to do so by police on scene.

    B. requested by patient.

    C. it interferes with airway management.

    D. it is longer than 12 inches.

51. An EMT must check which of the following when administering pharmaceuticals?

    A. Temperature of drug

    B. Contraindications

    C. Side effects

    D. Expiration date

52. Your patient is experiencing severe respiratory difficulty due to pulmonary edema. In which of the following positions would you expect to see this patient?

    A. Semi-Fowler position

    B. Trendelenburg position

    C. Tripod position

    D. Reverse Fowler position

53. The contraction of the ventricles produces the _____ pressure in the arteries.

    A. diastolic

    B. systolic

    C. arterial

    D. static

54. On a cold winter day, you respond to a local pond for an ice fisherman who fell through the ice. You arrive on scene and you observe a male lying supine in cold and wet clothes; the patient has no pulse or respirations. A scuba diver advises that your patient has been underwater for the 30 minutes it took the diver to suit up and effect the rescue. You should next

    A. pronounce the patient dead.

    B. immediately begin CPR.

    C. place the patient in the truck, remove his wet clothes, and begin to warm him.

    D. request an ALS intercept.

55. You are dispatched to a local health club for a male with difficulty breathing. You respond emergently and arrive on scene. The scene is safe and you are wearing suitable precautions. You observe a 30-year-old male patient with obvious dyspnea who is pale and mildly diaphoretic. He has a history of asthma, blood pressure of 150/80, pulse of 110, and respiratory rate of 24. His pulse oximetry saturation is 88% on room air. Which of the following oxygen delivery devices should you apply?

    A. Nasal cannula

    B. Simple face mask

    C. Bag-valve mask

    D. Non-rebreather mask

56. In the scenario in question 55, what flow rate will you set your oxygen regulator to?

    A. 4 liters per minute

    B. 10 liters per minute

    C. 15 liters per minute

    D. 20 liters per minute

57. Which of the following is NOT a landmark for a lung field you would auscultate in question 55?

    A. Anterior midclavicular

    B. Posterior base

    C. Inferior vena cava

    D. Right midaxillary

58. Which of the following foods are highly suspect in anaphylaxis?

    A. Nuts

    B. Seafood

    C. Eggs

    D. All of the above

59. Which of the following is NOT a classic symptom of a heart attack?

    A. Chest pain

    B. Dyspnea

    C. Denial

    D. Headache

60. The beginning of obstetrical labor is the

    A. discharge of the placenta.

    B. fertilization of the ovum.

    C. discharge of the cervical mucus plug.

    D. rupture of the amniotic sac.

61. Which of the following is useful in absorbing toxins in the stomach?

    A. Activated charcoal

    B. Ipecac syrup

    C. Oxygen

    D. Aspirin

62. Labor concludes with the delivery of the

    A. baby.

    B. placenta.

    C. umbilical cord.

    D. amniotic fluid.

63. You are dispatched to a call for chest pains. You respond emergently, the scene is safe, and you are wearing protective equipment. Your patient is a female in her sixties, seated at the kitchen table. She is guarding her chest with one hand and tells you she has crushing chest pain of sudden onset. She has a history of cardiac problems and is currently on nitroglycerine paste and Cardizem™. Her pulse is weak and thready. Which of the following drugs should you NOT administer?

    A. Aspirin

    B. NTG

    C. Epinephrine

    D. Oxygen

64. The preferred method of ventilating a patient in respiratory arrest in the prehospital setting is a

    A. manual ventilator.

    B. face mask.

    C. BVM.

    D. BVM with oxygen reservoir.

65. You are dispatched to a local restaurant for a man down. You arrive on scene and observe a male in full cardiac and respiratory arrest. You and your partner perform CPR for 2 minutes and then convert his heart rhythm with the AED; his pulse is 65 and blood pressure 90/60. After 2 minutes, he begins to have spontaneous respirations and his gag reflex returns, so you remove the oropharyngeal airway. You finish your assessment and begin transport to the nearest emergency department 15 minutes away. At 10 minutes from the hospital, he suddenly lapses into unconsciousness and again has no pulse or spontaneous respirations. Your next procedure should be which of the following?

    A. Begin chest compressions

    B. Begin rescue breathing

    C. Shock with the AED

    D. Request an ALS intercept

66. You are dispatched to a residence for an unconscious male. You respond emergently with suitable precautions and the scene is safe. You find a male subject lying on the kitchen floor with spontaneous respirations and carotid and radial pulses. He is conscious and responsive to verbal stimuli with a patent airway and no difficulty swallowing. You take his blood sugar with a glucometer and he has a blood sugar of 45. He is probably suffering from

    A. postictal seizure.

    B. hypoglycemia.

    C. hyperglycemia.

    D. hypovolemia.

67. The patient in question 66 should be given

    A. insulin.

    B. epinephrine.

    C. glucose.

    D. nitroglycerin.

68. Presentation of the cord from the vagina before delivery of the baby is called

    A. presenting cord.

    B. prolapsed cord.

    C. breech cord.

    D. premature cord.

69. You are dispatched to a local clinic for a child convulsing. You respond emergently wearing suitable precautions and arrive on scene. The nurse on scene advises that the mother brought her 2-year-old male child in for not feeling well and as she began to examine him, he began to seize. His vital signs are BP 100/60, pulse rate of 80, respirations of 18 prior to the seizure, and a rectal temperature of 105°F. You suspect the patient is having a _____ seizure.

    A. tonic/clonic

    B. postictal

    C. febrile

    D. anaphylactic

70. Which of the following indicates the normal blood glucose range in adults?

    A. 0–40 mg/dL

    B. 40–80 mg/dL

    C. 80–120 mg/dL

    D. 120–160 mg/dL

71. Another term for heart attack is

    A. myocardial infarction.

    B. congestive heart failure.

    C. mitral valve defect.

    D. left bundle branch block.

72. You are dispatched to a call for a possible allergic reaction. You are directed to a restaurant table where a male in his twenties is clutching his throat in severe respiratory distress. His partner tells you that he is allergic to nuts and nut products, but he has not had anything other than grilled steak with sautéed vegetables. Which drug do you want to administer following your initial assessment?

    A. Benadryl 50mg tablet

    B. Epinephrine 0.3 mg intramuscular

    C. Nitroglycerin spray sublingual

    D. Oxygen 2–6 lpm via non-rebreather

73. You and your partner arrive on scene of a female having a seizure. When you enter the room, you witness the patient's muscles tensing up and remaining rigid. What is this period of the seizure called?

    A. Tonic

    B. Clonic

    C. Generalized

    D. Postictal

74. A motor vehicle accident in which one vehicle strikes another broadside is also referred to as a _____ crash.

    A. front-end

    B. rear-end

    C. T-Bone

    D. rollover

75. You are dispatched to a local residence for a female acting strangely. You respond emergently wearing suitable precautions and arrive on scene simultaneously with the police. The house is extremely cold inside, and the patient is a female in her sixties wearing heavy clothing. She responds to your questions in a faint, intelligible voice and as you feel her neck for a carotid pulse, she is cold to the touch. Your treatment of this patient should include all of the following EXCEPT:

    A. Placing the patient in a warm environment

    B. Applying heat packs to the groin, axillary, and cervical regions

    C. Advising the patient to drink hot coffee

    D. Removing any possible wet clothing

76. The blood component that carries the antibodies the body uses to fight infection is/are

    A. hemoglobin.

    B. leukocytes.

    C. plasma.

    D. platelets.

77. You are dispatched to a residence for a patient unconscious. You respond emergently and arrive on scene. The scene is safe, and you are wearing universal precautions. The firefighters on the scene advise that they have removed the victim from his garage where his car was running. The patient has labored breathing and his face is cyanotic, but his lips and tongue are bright red. Which poison should you suspect?

    A. Carbon dioxide

    B. Carbon monoxide

    C. Gasoline

    D. Narcotic overdose

78. To which of the following treatment facilities would you transport the patient in question 77?

    A. Nearest level I trauma center

    B. Nearest emergency department

    C. Nearest level III trauma center

    D. Nearest facility with a hyperbaric chamber

79. On a hot summer day, you are dispatched to a road race site for a runner down. You respond emergently and arrive on scene to find a 25-year-old male lying unconscious on his back in his running clothes. He skin is red, dry, and very hot to the touch. His pulse is 120, respirations are 20, and blood pressure is 100/60. Which condition should you suspect?

    A. Heat cramps

    B. Heat exhaustion

    C. Heatstroke

    D. Heat overdose

80. Which should you immediately do for the patient in question 79?

    A. Transport priority

    B. Request an ALS intercept

    C. Administer oxygen 6 lpm via nasal cannula

    D. Transfer the patient to a cooler location and apply wet cloths to his head

81. Which of the following best defines a phobia?

   A. A feeling of sadness or worthlessness

   B. An alternate feeling of euphoria and depression

   C. An irrational fear

   D. A mistrust of everyone and everything

82. Tuberculosis is an example of a(n) _____ pathogen.

   A. airborne

   B. bloodborne

   C. fluidborne

   D. stillborn

83. Which of the following poisons could be vomited without danger?

   A. Bleach

   B. Kerosene

   C. Alcohol

   D. Ammonia

84. You are dispatched to a person in the water at a local reservoir. You respond emergently and arrive on scene before the police and fire units and observe a male yelling for help 100 yards from shore. You should immediately

   A. jump into the water and swim to the victim.

   B. check and see if there is a boat nearby that you can use to row to the victim.

   C. throw a life preserver to the victim.

   D. advise dispatch that you will need a rescue boat.

85. The EMT should ask the patient to do which of the following prior to administration of a bronchodilator?

   A. Hold his breath for 5 seconds

   B. Exhale deeply

   C. Inhale rapidly three times

   D. Pant

86. You are dispatched to the scene of a 12-year-old female who has been struck by a car in her neighborhood. Police on scene are unable to reach her parents. What gives you the ability to treat the girl?

   A. Explicit consent

   B. *In loco parentis*

   C. Informed consent

   D. Refusal of consent

87. You respond for a female who is having a behavioral emergency. The patient is not able to leave her house until she checks each door five times to make sure it is locked properly. This demonstrates which of the following types of behavior?

   A. Schizophrenia

   B. Psychosis

   C. OCD

   D. Impulse control disorder

88. Which of the following is the most common mental illness experience in the United States?

   A. Depression

   B. Manic-depressive illness

   C. Obsessive-compulsive disorder

   D. Bipolar mood disorder

89. At which stage of hypothermia does loss of consciousness normally occur?

   A. Mild

   B. Moderate

   C. Severe

   D. Irreversible

90. Most behavioral emergency calls are

   A. violent.

   B. nonviolent.

   C. exaggerated.

   D. wrongly dispatched.

91. Which of the following obstetrical conditions usually presents with painless, bright red bleeding?

    A. Abruptio placenta

    B. Multipara

    C. Placenta previa

    D. Supine hypotensive syndrome

92. APGAR scores are taken at 1 minute and _____ minutes postpartum.

    A. 2

    B. 5

    C. 10

    D. 20

93. The normal respiratory rate for an adult is

    A. 6–12 times per minute.

    B. 12–20 times per minute.

    C. 15–25 times per minute.

    D. 20–40 times per minute.

94. The heart contains _____ chambers.

    A. 1

    B. 2

    C. 3

    D. 4

95. Which of the following is the primary effect of chronic bronchitis on the airway?

    A. Failure of the hemoglobin to be able to carry oxygen

    B. Increased mucus production in the bronchial tree

    C. Increased bronchial dilation

    D. Decreased carbon dioxide production

96. What is the minimum number of people required to safely restrain a violent patient in 4-point soft restraints?

    A. 5

    B. 3

    C. 4

    D. 2

97. In which of the following situations should a police escort be used with EMT transport?

    A. Transport of a critical patient

    B. Transport of a mother and child postpartum

    C. Unfamiliarity with the location of the hospital

    D. Transport of a police officer injured in the line of duty

98. The normal gestation period for a human fetus is

    A. 12 weeks.

    B. 24 weeks.

    C. 40 weeks.

    D. 52 weeks.

99. The liquid component of the blood is called

    A. hemoglobin.

    B. leukocytes.

    C. plasma.

    D. platelets.

100. Obstetrical crowning is when

    A. the mother's amniotic sac ruptures.

    B. the baby's head becomes visible in the birth canal.

    C. labor pains are less than 5 minutes apart and last longer than 1 minute.

    D. the baby cries for the first time.

101. How many vertebrae make up the spinal column?

    A. 33

    B. 23

    C. 45

    D. 29

102. A patient who presents with hyperthermia, erratic behavior, super strength, and a history of illegal drug usage is most likely suffering from

    A. bipolar disorder.

    B. excited delirium.

    C. schizophrenia.

    D. panic disorder.

103. You are dispatched to a call for a "possible heart attack" to a residence along with an ALS rescue that is 10 minutes out. You respond emergently and arrive on scene 4 minutes after being dispatched. The scene is safe and you are wearing appropriate universal precautions. You observe a male in his seventies lying supine on the living room floor, cyanotic, with his eyes open. You open his airway and note that he is not breathing. You administer two breaths, which inflate his lungs. You check for a carotid pulse and there is none. You advise your partner to begin chest compressions. What is your next step?

    A. Continue rescue breathing and compressions pending arrival of ALS

    B. Place 15 lpm NRB

    C. Apply the AED and follow the directions

    D. After 1 minute of CPR, place the patient on a backboard and transport priority

104. Which of the following vehicles has the right of way over an ambulance?

    A. Police car with flashing lights operating

    B. Fire truck with flashing lights operating

    C. School bus with flashing lights operating

    D. Utility truck with flashing yellow lights operating

105. The ulna is located in the

    A. lower arm.

    B. lower leg.

    C. chest.

    D. face.

106. You are dispatched to a female in labor. You observe a female in her twenties lying in bed with her knees drawn up and her upper body supported by pillows in a semi-Fowler position. She advises you that this is her third pregnancy, that her water has broken, and that the pains are less than a minute apart. You examine her vaginal area, and as she experiences another contraction you see the top of the baby's head in the birth canal. You should next

    A. prepare for immediate delivery.

    B. place the mother on the stretcher left lateral recumbent and transport priority to the nearest obstetrical unit.

    C. tie the mother's legs together to slow delivery while you do a full assessment.

    D. boil water.

107. In the scenario in question 106, the next contraction delivers the baby's head. You notice the cord wrapped around the baby's neck. You should next

    A. clamp the cord.

    B. place two fingers between the cord and the baby's neck.

    C. cut the cord.

    D. request an ALS intercept.

108. In the scenario in question 106, after the baby is delivered you notice that she is not breathing. You should next

    A. begin CPR.

    B. suction with a bulb syringe.

    C. suction with the portable suction unit.

    D. slap the baby's bottom.

109. If an EMT makes an error while writing a paper PCR narrative, which of the following should be done?

    A. Disregard the error and continue with the narrative

    B. Destroy the document

    C. Cross out the error, write a correction, and date and sign the correction

    D. Write a new narrative and staple it to the old narrative

110. Why are the bottom two ribs called floating ribs?

    A. They are not connected to the sternum.

    B. They are not connected to any other bony structure.

    C. They are suspended in fluid.

    D. They are not really ribs.

111. All calls for behavioral emergencies should also have a(n)

    A. ALS intercept.

    B. police response.

    C. second rescue.

    D. fire department response.

112. What is the maximum APGAR score?

    A. 5

    B. 8

    C. 10

    D. 12

113. A patient has a blood glucose level of 45 mg/dL. This is considered what type of emergency?

    A. Hyperglycemic

    B. Diabetic ketoacidosis

    C. Hypoglycemic

    D. Insulin shock

114. Victims of sexual assault should be initially assessed and treated by

    A. EMTs of the same gender if possible.

    B. police officers trained in sexual assault.

    C. registered nurses.

    D. rape crisis counselors.

115. Which route describes placing medication in the cheek mucosal area?

    A. Oral

    B. Sublingual

    C. Buccal

    D. Tympanic

116. Which of the following incidents are the most common EMS trauma call?

    A. Falls

    B. Shootings

    C. Stabbings

    D. Motor vehicle accidents

117. In treatment of severe trauma, what is the recognized time standard from injury to the operating room?

    A. 30 minutes

    B. 60 minutes

    C. 180 minutes

    D. 240 minutes

118. How many liters of blood are in the average adult human's circulatory system?

    A. 2–3

    B. 3–4

    C. 4–5

    D. 5–6

119. The most common cause of seizures in the infant population is

    A. epilepsy.
    B. high fever.
    C. poisoning.
    D. mother's use of illegal drugs while pregnant.

120. You are dispatched to a residence for a man with a lacerated arm. You respond emergently and arrive on scene wearing suitable precautions; the police are on scene. Your patient is lying on the ground behind the house with a series of lacerations around his lower arm. He is bleeding profusely with a steady flow but does not appear to be spurting. He is intoxicated and belligerent. You attempt to control the bleeding with pressure bandages but he continues to hemorrhage. Which procedure is the next best option?

    A. Hemostatic agent
    B. Tourniquet
    C. Pressure bandage
    D. Oxygen at 15 lpm NRB

121. The most common cause of dyspnea in the infant is

    A. foreign bodies.
    B. mucus.
    C. congenital birth defects.
    D. SIDS.

122. What is the most desirable characteristic the EMT wants in a dressing?

    A. Size
    B. Shape
    C. Sterility
    D. Elasticity

123. Which of the following is NOT true as it pertains to refusal to treat or transport?

    A. The treatment and transport options must be explained.
    B. The consequences of refusal must be explained.
    C. The patient may not change their mind once they sign a refusal.
    D. The signature of the patient must be witnessed by a disinterested third party.

124. You are dispatched to a motor vehicle accident on the highway. You respond emergently and arrive on scene wearing suitable BSI gear. The police and fire department are on scene. Your patient is a male lying next to his wrecked car. He has been collared and spine boarded by the fire department. He is responsive to painful stimuli with vital signs of BP 100/60, pulse of 120, respirations of 18. He is pale and clammy. Your treatment of this patient should include all of the following EXCEPT:

    A. Focused trauma assessment en route
    B. Prevention of heat loss
    C. High flow oxygen
    D. Fowler position

125. Which of the following is NOT a type of open wound?

    A. Abrasion
    B. Incision
    C. Bruising
    D. Laceration

126. One of the side effects of nitroglycerin tablets is

    A. hypotension.
    B. hypertension.
    C. diaphoresis.
    D. tachypnea.

127. Wounds to which of the following anatomical areas should be treated with occlusive dressings?

    A. Head

    B. Neck

    C. Abdomen

    D. Genitals

128. You are dispatched along with the fire department to a report of a person on fire behind a residence. You respond emergently and arrive simultaneously with the fire department. A woman tells you her husband was lighting his charcoal grill with gasoline and there was an explosion. The patient is a male subject who is conscious, alert, and oriented times three. He states he was trying to light the grill when the gasoline exploded. He denies any dyspnea. The physical exam reveals second-degree burns to both arms and there is no other part of the body burned. What percentage of the patient's body is burned?

    A. 9%

    B. 18%

    C. 27%

    D. 20%

129. In the scenario in question 128, what priority is this patient?

    A. Non-priority

    B. Critical

    C. Moderate

    D. Fatal

130. Naloxone is a drug given for the following drug and in what dosage?

    A. Heroin OD, 2 mg total IN

    B. Opioid OD, 6 mg total IN

    C. LSD OD, 2 mg total IN

    D. NSAID OD, 4 mg total IN

131. You are dispatched to the high school football field for a player injured. You respond emergently and arrive on scene wearing suitable precautions. The coach advises you that he suspects the player has a fractured fibula. The patient is conscious, alert, and oriented times three, and his only complaint is severe pain in his lower leg. When considering what type of splint to apply, where must the suspected fracture site always be splinted?

    A. Below the injury

    B. Above and below the injury

    C. Above the injury

    D. Over the injury

132. In the scenario in question 131, which situation would lead you to attempt to reduce the broken bone?

    A. Lower leg fracture

    B. Absence of distal pulse

    C. Hypovolemic shock

    D. Femur fracture

133. The letter "M" in the acronym SAMPLE stands for

    A. menstrual period.

    B. medications.

    C. most active symptom.

    D. movement.

134. The epiglottis in a pediatric patient is _____ in the airway than in an adult patient.

    A. more sensitive

    B. higher

    C. lower

    D. more anterior

135. In which of the following injury situations should you apply a cervical collar?

    A. Head trauma secondary to a rear-end motor vehicle collision

    B. Fall from a garage roof

    C. Neck pain as a result of a football injury

    D. All of the above

136. The narrative section of the prehospital care report should include all of the following EXCEPT:

    A. What the patient looked like on EMS arrival

    B. What medications the patient is currently taking

    C. The vital signs of the patient

    D. The patient's next of kin

137. You are dispatched to a two-car motor vehicle accident and respond emergently. You arrive on scene, the scene is safe, and you are wearing appropriate precautions. Your patient is in a vehicle that was struck broadside by another vehicle traveling at a high rate of speed. He was not restrained and is complaining of dyspnea. His shirt is ripped and bloody and you notice that he has an open wound that is gurgling and foaming. This patient is most at risk for

    A. hypovolemic shock.

    B. pneumothorax.

    C. subdural hematoma.

    D. myocardial infarction

138. Patients with open abdominal injuries are at greater risk for which of the following?

    A. Hypertension

    B. Infection

    C. Sudden cardiac death

    D. Peritonitis

139. A patient aged 8 months is defined as a(n)

    A. neonate.

    B. toddler.

    C. infant.

    D. preschooler.

140. If a tourniquet is applied to control bleeding, at what point should it be loosened?

    A. Every 5 minutes

    B. Every 10 minutes

    C. Every 15 minutes

    D. At the hospital

141. You are called to respond with police to a local residence for a psychological evaluation. You respond emergently with suitable precautions, and when you arrive the police have secured the scene. A male in his thirties is pacing around the room anxiously. He is not cooperative or responsive to your questions, and the police advise that his psychiatrist has requested his transport to the nearest emergency department for medical evaluation prior to admittance to the psychiatric facility. As the patient hears this, he attacks the police officer but is quickly subdued. The police officer advises you that the patient's psychiatrist has approved the use of restraints. What is the most proper way to restrain this patient?

    A. Prone with hands behind the back and ankles drawn up to the wrists

    B. Supine with hands behind the back and ankles secured to the stretcher

    C. Supine with both hands and ankles secured to the stretcher

    D. Prone with handcuffs attached to both the wrists and ankles

142. You are dispatched to a local nursing home for a patient who has fallen. You respond emergently with suitable precautions and the scene is safe. You find an 82-year-old female lying supine on the floor, conscious and alert, complaining of pain to her hip. You note that her right leg is rotated outward. What splinting device should you use?

    A. Traction splint

    B. Pelvic binder

    C. Padded board splint

    D. Backboard

143. Which of the following types of bleeding is the most severe?

    A. Capillary

    B. Venous

    C. Arteriole

    D. Arterial

144. Aspirin is indicated for which of the following conditions in EMS protocols?

    A. Headache

    B. Chest pain

    C. Abdominal pain

    D. Leg and arm pain

145. Which of the following persons are NOT allowed to routinely access a prehospital care report?

    A. The patient

    B. The receiving physician

    C. The police

    D. The EMT who wrote the report

146. What is the book used to identify hazardous materials?

    A. EEG book

    B. ERG book

    C. ENT book

    D. EKG book

147. Which of the following pregnancies will normally have a longer labor period?

    A. First

    B. Second

    C. Third

    D. Fourth

148. At the scene of a motor vehicle accident, the ambulance should be parked so as to

    A. remain downhill and downwind from the scene.

    B. protect the scene.

    C. be able to load the patient into the back doors.

    D. not obstruct the police investigation.

149. Once the cervix is fully dilated and the baby "drops" into the birth canal, this is referred to as the

    A. first stage of labor.

    B. second stage of labor.

    C. third stage of labor.

    D. fourth stage of labor.

150. Which of the following is an example of implied consent?

    A. Patient who agrees to be transported to the emergency department

    B. Pediatric patient whose parent allows him to be treated and transported

    C. Unconscious patient

    D. Patient who is diagnosed with schizophrenia and refuses transport

Answer Key

1.	**C**	21.	**C**	41.	**C**	61.	**A**	81.	**C**
2.	**C**	22.	**D**	42.	**D**	62.	**B**	82.	**A**
3.	**D**	23.	**D**	43.	**B**	63.	**C**	83.	**C**
4.	**C**	24.	**D**	44.	**D**	64.	**D**	84.	**D**
5.	**D**	25.	**A**	45.	**B**	65.	**A**	85.	**B**
6.	**A**	26.	**D**	46.	**D**	66.	**B**	86.	**B**
7.	**C**	27.	**D**	47.	**D**	67.	**C**	87.	**C**
8.	**D**	28.	**C**	48.	**A**	68.	**B**	88.	**A**
9.	**D**	29.	**B**	49.	**A**	69.	**C**	89.	**C**
10.	**C**	30.	**C**	50.	**C**	70.	**C**	90.	**B**
11.	**C**	31.	**A**	51.	**D**	71.	**A**	91.	**C**
12.	**D**	32.	**B**	52.	**C**	72.	**B**	92.	**B**
13.	**A**	33.	**C**	53.	**B**	73.	**A**	93.	**B**
14.	**D**	34.	**B**	54.	**B**	74.	**C**	94.	**D**
15.	**B**	35.	**C**	55.	**D**	75.	**C**	95.	**B**
16.	**C**	36.	**A**	56.	**C**	76.	**B**	96.	**D**
17.	**B**	37.	**D**	57.	**C**	77.	**B**	97.	**C**
18.	**C**	38.	**B**	58.	**D**	78.	**D**	98.	**C**
19.	**A**	39.	**C**	59.	**D**	79.	**C**	99.	**C**
20.	**B**	40.	**D**	60.	**C**	80.	**D**	100.	**B**

(Continued)

101. **A**	121. **B**	141. **C**
102. **B**	122. **C**	142. **D**
103. **C**	123. **C**	143. **D**
104. **C**	124. **D**	144. **B**
105. **A**	125. **C**	145. **C**
106. **A**	126. **A**	146. **B**
107. **B**	127. **B**	147. **A**
108. **B**	128. **B**	148. **B**
109. **C**	129. **C**	149. **A**
110. **A**	130. **A**	150. **C**
111. **B**	131. **B**	
112. **C**	132. **B**	
113. **C**	133. **B**	
114. **A**	134. **B**	
115. **C**	135. **D**	
116. **D**	136. **D**	
117. **B**	137. **B**	
118. **D**	138. **B**	
119. **B**	139. **C**	
120. **A**	140. **D**	

Answers and Explanations

1. C

Any dispatch to a call with violence involved, such as a gunshot wound, must be secured by police prior to EMS involvement. The other calls give no indication of being unsafe scenes.

2. C

The path of blood flow goes from the heart to the aorta to the arteries to the arterioles to the capillaries to the venules to the veins to the vena cavae to the heart.

3. D

The very young and very old are at greater risk for hypothermia.

4. C

Crying may be a response to the depressive stage of grief, but is not a stage of grief. Denial, anger, and acceptance are among the five stages. The missing stages from this list are depression and bargaining.

5. D

The zygomatic bones are the cheekbones. Zygomatic fractures are very common among males age twenties and thirties, often as a result of blunt trauma.

6. A

The Emergency Medical Treatment and Active Labor Act (EMTALA) was enacted by Congress in 1986. It ensures public access to emergency services regardless of one's ability to pay and also prevents hospitals from sending their patients to other hospitals because of the patient's financial status. The White Paper Act (B) was a paper published in 1966 addressing the inadequacy of prehospital emergency medical care. HIPAA (C) was created to protect the privacy of health care information. There is no such act as the Medical Practice Act of 1988 (D).

7. C

Helicopters are dangerous vehicles, and they have safety rules. Do not approach from the uphill side because of the danger of the rotors. Do not approach from the rear because of the tail rotor. Do not approach until instructed by a helicopter crew member so that the patient loading can be coordinated safely. Not approaching the helicopter (D) may be impractical due to patient care concerns.

8. D

(A), (B), and (C) are all significant in conducting patient assessment. A patient's medical insurance is not a consideration in treating emergency patients.

9. D

(A), (B), and (C) are all components of the Glasgow Coma Scale (GCS), which describes a patient's level of consciousness after a traumatic brain injury, with best motor response, best verbal response, and eye opening. Grimace response is not part of the measurement.

10. C

In order to prove negligence, there must be four elements: duty, breach of duty, proximate cause, and harm caused. Simple negligence typically defines careless mistakes or inattention. Gross negligence defines conscious or willful disregard of the need to use reasonable care.

11. C

Superior refers to an upper region, so the head is considered superior to the chest, while the chest would be considered inferior to the head. Anterior is the front, and posterior is the back.

12. D

The "A" in DCAP-BTLS stands for abrasions.

13. A

Exam questions about the number of vertebrae in each section of the spine are common. There are five vertebrae in the lumbar section. For review, the cervical section of the spine has 7 vertebrae, the thoracic 12, the lumbar 5, the sacral 5, and the coccyx 4.

14. D

Loss of spontaneity is not a characteristic symptom of PTSD. The other answer choices are all symptoms of PTSD, and if they last longer than a few days, the EMT should be referred for professional help.

15. B

A baby's ability to make a facial expression ("to grimace") is indicative of its ability to function in the outside world. A grimace response or reflex irritability describes a response to stimulation, such as a mild pinch. None of the other answer choices are indicators in the APGAR score. Grating refers to rubbing of two organs together, guarding is when one protects a portion of the body with one's hands, and gurgling is the sound one makes when there is fluid in the oropharynx.

16. C

Unless contraindicated by some other condition, people in their third trimester of pregnancy should be transported on their left side. This will prevent the weight of the child from compressing the vena cavae and causing circulatory problems, which could lead to impairment of consciousness and other complications. Trendelenburg is when the legs are elevated to help combat hypotension, and Fowler position is seated upright.

17. B

Because the patient has already expressed the desire to harm himself to a public safety official, the patient must be evaluated by a physician. If the patient refuses to go, the police may have to place the patient in protective custody to have him transported to the hospital.

18. C

The patient is not exhibiting a behavior that requires an overly aggressive response, such as tackling her or wrestling her to the stretcher. Speak to her gently. She is having delusions, and it is not wise to acknowledge them and "shake Mr. Nureyev's hand." She might protest when you tell her that Mr. Nureyev is not there dancing with

her, but your confidence and gentle demeanor should win her over and help her to cooperate.

19. A

Neonates have higher pulse rates and respiratory rates than infants. There is no change in regularity between neonates and infants.

20. B

Most EMTs are injured while treating injured patients at motor vehicle accidents and thus should be more alert to the dangers posed by being on the streets and highways. The other situations also present dangers of which the EMT must be aware, but the MVA is the leading cause of injury.

21. C

Veins carry deoxygenated blood toward the heart. The vessels that carry blood away from the heart are the arteries.

22. D

The three types of muscles are voluntary, involuntary, and cardiac. There is no such thing as a regulatory muscle.

23. D

SAMPLE stands for Signs and symptoms, Allergies, Medications, Pertinent past history, Last oral intake, and Events leading up to this situation. Pulse rate is a vital sign.

24. D

Communication equipment should be checked at the start of every shift. No self-respecting EMT would like to find out 2 hours into the shift that his radio was not working and that calls were missed.

25. A

Before anything else is done, you must be certain that the scene is safe to operate in. Universal precautions should already be in place prior to arrival on scene.

26. D

While all of these injuries may be possible with this type of scenario, the most serious injury would be spinal damage, particularly in the cervical region (D). A bulls-eye pattern indicates that the patient struck his head with a significant amount of force to the windshield, which would have both an direct and indirect force directed down his spinal cord, which may damage vertebrae along the way.

27. D

Once the scene is determined to be safe and the EMT is wearing proper precautions, the EMT must assess the level of consciousness.

28. C

(A), (B), and (D) are all descriptions of levels of consciousness.

29. B

Perfusion refers to the percentage of oxygen that a red blood cell can carry to the cells and is measured by the use of the pulse oximeter. This is a vital sign for determining how efficiently the lungs are transferring oxygen to the red blood cells and how well the heart is pumping those cells throughout the body. Basic EMS does not have the diagnostic capabilities to determine the other answers.

30. C

Core body temperature 91°F indicates mild hypothermia. Body temperature 82.4–89.6°F indicates moderate hypothermia, and body temperature less than 82.4°F indicates severe hypothermia. Irreversible hypothermia (D) is not considered a stage of hypothermia.

31. A

This patient would benefit from an ALS intervention considering his underlying medical problem and weakened lungs. His pulse is weak and thready, and he is unresponsive. He is indeed a "priority" patient, but priority transport (B) would require much more time than ALS (30 min versus 15 min). Also, ALS can perform more advanced airway and cardiac management. (C) would be used only if the assessment gave some indication that his level of consciousness was caused by an allergic reaction. A helicopter (D) is not appropriate since the amount of time spent taking off and landing would delay arrival at the emergency department.

32. B

OPQRST stands for Onset, Provocation, Quality, Radiation, Severity, and Time. This question also reinforces the need to read the question carefully, since the words *quality* and *quantity* are very similar.

33. C

Good patient assessment requires that vital signs and assessment observations be checked and tended every 5 minutes, since patient condition can change very rapidly.

34. B

(A) and (D) describe a direct force injury. (C) describes a pathological fracture.

35. C

The mnemonic DCAP-BTLS is used in the focused assessment of a trauma patient and stands for Deformity, Contusions, Abrasions, Punctures, Burns, Tenderness, Lacerations, and Swelling.

36. A

The midaxillary line runs through the underarm of the patient, dividing the anterior plane from the posterior plane.

37. D

The proper order for securing a cervical spine is as follows. First, a focused assessment to find any bleeding, step-offs, bones out-of-place, tracheal deviation, JVD, pain, or abnormal sensations. Next is placement of a properly sized c-collar (D). After that, the partner who is holding c-spine must not let go (even with the collar on) until the person is fully secured to a long or short backboarding device. If using a long backboard, then head blocks (A) are appropriate, but that is not what this question is asking. There is no mention of a femur fracture, so hare traction (B) is incorrect. While the patient may require oxygen, nothing here states that, so an NRB mask is not appropriate.

38. B

The Good Samaritan Act was passed to encourage people to render aid by minimizing the liability for such acts.

39. C

While 5 minutes is the standard, vital signs should be retaken anytime there is any change in the patient's condition. Changes in the patient's condition will only be noted if the patient's ongoing assessment is constant and not just at a predetermined interval.

40. D

AVPU stands for Alert, Verbal, Pain, Unresponsive, and is used to assign a level of consciousness to a patient. A patient who does not awaken when yelled at and doesn't respond to a vigorous rubbing of his sternum is considered unresponsive.

41. C

Patient confidentiality laws mandate that the patient's name and specific medical information be kept confidential. Broadcasting a patient's name over the radio, which is monitored, would be a violation of this confidentiality. (A) and (B) would be important information in responding to a call.

42. D

While some reports do have spaces for emergency contacts, this information is not required for the patient care report.

43. B

When bandaging an eye injury, you must cover both eyes to prevent the sympathetic movement of the uninjured eye from causing further injury to the injured eye. In the absence of other injuries, there is no need to bandage the entire upper head.

44. D

All states mandate reporting by medical providers to the appropriate state agency if they become aware of child abuse. Some states also require reporting of sexual abuse, elder abuse, and spousal abuse, but that is not yet universal. Alcohol abuse (D) could require multiple visits by emergency responders (alcoholics are prone to self-harm behaviors, altered mental status, falls with subsequent injuries, or driving while under the influence), but this is considered a regular type of medical emergency and would not require mandatory reporting.

45. B

Once the cord ceases pulsing and the baby is breathing on her own, it is safe to cut the cord. If the cord is cut before the pulsing has ceased, there is a danger of the mother exsanguinating (bleeding). In waiting until the placenta is delivered, there is no increased danger to the mother or neonate, nor would waiting to arrive at the hospital be a problem. However, in order to properly treat the neonate, it would be easier to have her separated from the placenta.

46. D

Dropping blood pressure (A), excessive thirst (B), and tachypnea (C) are all symptoms of hypovolemic shock, along with tachycardia, or fast heart rate. Hypertension (D) is not seen in shock.

47. D

A competent and conscious patient may refuse any medical procedure or transport.

48. A

The nasal cannula is a lightweight, easy-to-use device that provides 24–40% oxygen. It is given when patients are stable and when a low flow of oxygen is required. The simple face mask provides 35–55% oxygen. A patient who requires low-flow oxygen would most likely find the nasal cannula more comfortable than the face mask, since it requires only an insertion into the nose (as opposed to both the mouth and nose). The non-rebreather mask provides 90–100% oxygen; and the bag-valve mask provides nearly 100% oxygen.

49. A

SIDS normally occurs in the neonate and infant populations, although toddlers are also occasionally at risk.

50. C

An impaled object should never be removed unless it interferes with managing the airway or performing chest compressions.

51. D

The expiration date must always be checked. The other answers should also be checked, but answer choice (D), expiration date, is one of the 5 Rights to be checked in drug administration.

52. C

A patient with severe respiratory difficulty due to pulmonary edema would most likely present in the tripod position. A patient with respiratory difficulty due to pulmonary edema would not find any relief in the Trendelenburg position or the reverse Fowler position and would generally only find moderate relief in the semi-Fowler position.

53. B

The systolic pressure in the arteries occurs when the ventricles contract and force the blood through the circulatory system. Diastolic pressure occurs when the heart is relaxing between contractions. Arterial pressure is the general pressure in the arteries.

54. B

The patient may still be resuscitated, since his vital signs may have been suppressed by sudden immersion in cold water, a condition referred to as the mammalian diving reflex. EMS personnel cannot normally pronounce people dead, although state protocols do usually allow EMTs to assume death has occurred if certain signs and symptoms, such as rigor mortis and postmortem lividity, are present. You will want to warm the patient by cutting away his clothing and placing him in a warm truck, but your priority should be beginning CPR. You may request an ALS intercept, but it is imperative that basic life support begin immediately.

55. D

The patient is hypoxic and needs high-flow oxygen, and the device that will provide the most flow is the non-rebreather, which delivers between 90 and 100% oxygen to the patient. The other devices deliver less: the nasal cannula (A) delivers 24 to 40%, the simple face mask (B) 40 to 60%. A BVM would be inappropriate here as the patient is still alert and while his oxygen levels are low and concerning, his respiratory rate is not excessively high or low. A non-rebreather mask would be the best choice.

56. C

The maximum liter flow for the full non-rebreather is 15 liters per minute.

57. C

The inferior vena cava is a blood vessel that returns deoxygenated blood to the heart and has little to do with auscultation of breath sounds.

58. D

Any food product listed may be implicated in anaphylaxis, or allergic reaction.

59. D

All of the other answers, including denial, are symptoms of a myocardial infarction.

60. C

The first stage of labor begins when the mucus plug is discharged from the cervix. Labor ends following the delivery of the placenta, or afterbirth. Fertilization of the ovum is the beginning of gestation or pregnancy. The amniotic sac usually, but not always, ruptures during the first stage of labor after the mucus plug is discharged.

61. A

Activated charcoal is very effective at absorbing toxins in the stomach before they can be absorbed into the bloodstream. Ipecac (B) causes vomiting, oxygen (C) is used for respiratory problems, and aspirin (D) is an analgesic and in EMS is used only in the chest pain protocols.

62. B

Labor concludes with the delivery of the placenta.

63. C

Epinephrine is indicated in cardiac arrest, but not in the treatment of chest pain, nor is it in most BLS protocols. Aspirin (A) and oxygen (D) are always indicated in the treatment of sudden chest pain. Medical control may order nitroglycerin (B) if state protocols allow.

64. D

A bag-valve mask with an oxygen reservoir is the most effective method of ventilating a patient in the prehospital setting. A manual ventilator (A) is unwieldy in the prehospital setting, and a face mask (B) is not as effective in ventilating as a bag-valve mask. The oxygen reservoir also makes the percentage of oxygen much higher than the other prehospital devices do.

65. A

If an arrest reoccurs, compressions will need to be resumed due to lack of a pulse or breathing. Because he is not breathing on his own, (B) is inappropriate. Rescue breathing is used when a patient is breathing at inadequate rates on his own (ideally with the use of a simple face mask or BVM). An AED is a plausible answer; however, it would need to analyze the heart first before allowing the shock button to be pressed. ALS intercept is also a possibility, but the best answer is (A).

66. B

This patient is having a diabetic emergency caused by low blood sugar, or hypoglycemia. Normal blood sugar levels are 80–120 mg/dL. Postictal seizure (A) meets the symptoms except for the low blood sugar; hyperglycemia (C) is high blood sugar, which is definitely not the case here; and hypovolemia (D) would be caused by loss of blood volume, which is not suggested here.

67. C

The patient's blood sugar must be elevated. This is done by administering sugar, or glucose. Insulin (A) is not a drug that is indicated in this case. Epinephrine (B) is for an allergic reaction, and nitroglycerin (D) is for chest pain.

68. B

When the cord presents first, there is great danger that the cord will be compressed between the vaginal walls and the baby's head, cutting off circulation and oxygen to the baby. This is also technically a breech delivery, but "prolapsed cord" is the more correct terminology.

69. C

Most infant seizures are caused by a high temperature, or fever. Tonic/clonic (A) refers to the extremely jerky

movements of a full-blown seizure, postictal (B) is the state of unconsciousness that follows the tonic/clonic portion of the seizure, and anaphylactic (D) refers to allergic reaction.

70. C

Normal blood glucose ranges from 80–120 mg/dL in adult patients.

71. A

A heart attack occurs when a coronary artery is blocked and in turn a portion of the heart muscle becomes ischemic from lack of oxygen, or infarcts. The other answers are all cardiac conditions, but not literally a heart attack.

72. B

This patient is exhibiting symptoms of an allergic reaction and needs the immediate intervention of epinephrine, an intervention allowed to EMTs by many state protocols. Even if he has not knowingly ingested any known allergen, the food he has eaten may have been prepared with a nut product and this may be the cause. Oxygen (D) may be indicated, but not in low-flow amounts. Epinephrine is the best answer.

73. A

Tonic (A) is when the muscle becomes rigid and stays that way for a period of time, while clonic (B) is when the uncontrollable jerking happens. (C) is a type of seizure category, while (D) is the phase after a seizure occurs.

74. C

A vehicle struck broadside is referred to as a T-bone crash. All these crashes may be serious or fatal, but the best answer is T-bone.

75. C

Unless a medication in liquid form is to be given to the patient by mouth, most EMS systems do not allow for the administration of oral liquids such as hot coffee as part of patient care. The reason is that hot liquids could have unintended consequences. All of the other answer choices would be done to treat this patient's hypothermia.

76. B

Leukocytes, or white blood cells, are the body's primary mechanism for combating infection and disease. Hemoglobin is the protein that carries oxygen in blood. Plasma is the fluid part of blood. Platelets are what bind together to form clots.

77. B

The telltale sign of carbon-monoxide poisoning is bright red lips and tongue. Carbon dioxide (A) is not directly poisonous but can cause anoxia, since it displaces oxygen in the air; gasoline (C) is a petroleum distillate; and a narcotic overdose (D) will not cause red lips.

78. D

Carbon-monoxide poisoning is best treated by a hyperbaric chamber. Such a chamber forces oxygen into the hemoglobin under pressure and displaces the carbon monoxide. State protocols and medical control naturally dictate the proper course of action. A level I trauma center (A) has equipment and staff to deal with all cases of trauma, while a level III center (C) has minimal equipment and staff and will often stabilize a patient in preparation for transfer to a level I center.

79. C

The patient's condition indicates that his sweating mechanism has been compromised and his temperature is dangerously high. This condition is called heatstroke. Heat cramps (A) are muscle aches caused by hyperthermia, and heat exhaustion (B) is impaired consciousness brought on by hyperthermia, but without the disruption of the sweating mechanism.

80. D

This patient needs to be cooled immediately and then transported. Oxygen should be administered at whatever liters per minute are adequate per the patient's presentation and SpO2 level (a minimum of 94% should be the goal for proper oxygenation). An ALS intercept is a possibility, but the priority is to cool the patient down to prevent seizures, possible brain insult, and death.

81. C

Phobias are irrational fears. A feeling of sadness or worthlessness is often the result of clinical depression, the alternating feelings of euphoria and depression are symptomatic of bipolar disorder, and a mistrust of everyone and everything is paranoia.

82. A

Tuberculosis is transmitted by an airborne bacteria.

83. C

Alcohol (C) can be vomited without danger. The other answer choices can do more harm coming back through the esophagus than they caused going down. Vomiting caustic bleach or ammonia could severely damage the delicate and thin tissues of the esophagus. (Additionally, note that if mixed together, bleach and ammonia would cause a chemical reaction and toxic fumes, which should never be inhaled.) Vomiting kerosene or any other petroleum product could aspirate the product into the lungs.

84. D

The victim is too far to reach with a life preserver, and you should never attempt to swim to a victim unless you are confident in both your swimming ability and your ability to actually rescue a drowning person. While choice (B) is tempting, you cannot verify that the boat is safe to use or equipped as you would need. Choice (D) is correct, as rescue boat personnel are trained in both specialized equipment and water rescue techniques not typically part of entry-level EMS courses.

85. B

Prior to the administration of a bronchodilator, the EMT asks the patient to exhale deeply to remove as much air from the lungs as possible, and then to inhale the vapor deeply into the lungs for maximum effect.

86. B

In loco parentis (B) is the Latin term for "in place of parents" and is a type of implied consent. Explicit consent (A) is not a type of consent in EMS. Informed consent (C) is not appropriate, as the child is a minor and is unable to provide that type of consent for treatment. Refusal of consent (D) is not an option here.

87. C

Patients who lack the ability to resist a temptation or who cannot avoid acting on an impulse have an impulse control disorder. Obsessive-compulsive disorder (OCD) is a form of an impulse control disorder and typically involves repetitive actions, as exhibited by the patient here.

88. A

Depression is the leading cause of disability in people age 15–44, and it is the most common mental illness of the answer choices listed here. Anxiety disorders are not listed as an answer, but are the second most common mental illness in the United States.

89. C

Unconsciousness usually occurs in the severe stage of hypothermia. Mild hypothermia is marked by shivering as the body tries to raise its temperature. Moderate stage is when consciousness and judgment begin to become impaired and there is a loss of motor functions. In severe hypothermia, unconsciousness sets in and the extremities begin to freeze.

90. B

Most behavioral emergency calls are nonviolent, but the EMT must always be prepared to deal with violent patients.

91. C

Placenta previa usually presents with painless, bright red bleeding. Abruptio placenta (A) will present with severe pain and dark red bleeding. Multipara (B) simply means the patient has been pregnant multiple times. Supine hypotensive syndrome (D) does not present with bleeding.

92. B

APGAR scores are taken at 1 and 5 minutes postpartum, to check on the health of the baby and whether emergency care (oftentimes suctioning of the airways) is needed. The 1-minute score assesses the newborn's condition at 1 minute of life, i.e., heart rate, color, muscle tone. The 5-minute score reassesses those things a few minutes later.

93. B

Most texts give the normal adult respiratory rate as 12–20 times per minute. None of the other answers would be considered normal.

94. D

The four chambers are the left and right atria and the left and right ventricles.

95. B

The hallmark sign of chronic bronchitis is the excessive mucus production that occurs in the bronchial tree. Chronic bronchitis patients do not have a failure of the oxygen-carrying capacity of the hemoglobin, and there is an increase in carbon dioxide production. Because of the increased mucus production, the bronchioles will become constricted, not dilated.

96. D

Ideally, five people are needed: one person for each limb and one to apply the restraints. However, the minimum number needed is two.

97. C

Use of a police escort is not a common practice, and it has been statistically shown to be more hazardous than not using one. The reason is that citizen drivers likely don't realize that *both* a police car and ambulance are passing, and so pull back into traffic too early and cause congestion or even a collision. Use a police escort only when you are unfamiliar with the hospital and the GPS is not working.

98. C

The normal gestation period is 9 months from conception, or 40 weeks.

99. C

Plasma is the liquid part of the blood that carries the other components through the circulatory system. The other components are hemoglobin, or red blood cells; leukocytes, or white blood cells; and platelets.

100. B

Crowning is when the baby's head becomes visible. The mother's amniotic sac and the baby's crying have nothing to do with this term. Labor pains that are less than 5 minutes apart but longer than 1 minute are an indication that delivery is imminent.

101. A

There are a total of 33 vertebrae in the spinal column. There are 7 cervical, 12 thoracic, 5 lumbar, 5 fused sacrum, and 4 fused bones of the coccyx.

102. B

Excited delirium is the extreme overstimulation of the body and nervous system, typically caused by illegal drug usage. Bipolar disorder (A) is the same as manic-depressive syndrome. Schizophrenia (C) is a long-term mental disorder of a type involving a breakdown in the relation between thought, emotion, and behavior. Panic disorder (D) is when the patient becomes overly anxious about a situation that does not warrant that sort of response.

103. C

Application of the AED may diagnose a dysrhythmia, which may then be treated by a countershock and restore a normal heartbeat, or it may advise to continue CPR. Administration of epinephrine in this instance is an ALS intervention and since ALS has already been dispatched, you should maintain your patient with CPR pending their arrival, but your first step is to apply the AED.

104. C

A school bus with flashing lights has the right of way over all other vehicles, including ambulances. Police cars and fire trucks have the same rights of way as ambulances, but no additional privileges.

105. A

The ulna is one of the two bones in the lower arm.

106. A

Crowning is indicative of imminent delivery. Attempting to transport the mother at this point will result in delivery in the back of the ambulance. The legs should

never be tied together, as this will cause damage to both the mother and the baby. Boiling water is what you send anxious onlookers to get to keep them out of the way.

107. B

If the baby presents with the cord wrapped around the neck, you must either unwrap the cord or open the baby's airway by relieving the pressure of the cord around the neck. Clamping or cutting the cord will impair the circulation of the baby and may cause the mother to bleed out.

108. B

Immediately after delivery, the baby's mouth and nose should be suctioned with a bulb syringe to facilitate the baby's own breathing. A portable suction unit provides too much suction and could damage the baby's lungs. Slapping the baby's bottom may help stimulate spontaneous respirations, but you still need to clear the airway first. If the baby does not start breathing spontaneously, then begin CPR.

109. C

A PCR is a legal document, so changes may be made only by the person who is writing the narrative. The changes must be noticeable and documented, and are best made by crossing out (with a single line through the error) and then adding one's own initials and the current date in that same location. Disregarding the error (A) would compound the error by suggesting that it was the actual assessment or treatment given. Destroying the document (B) would break the serial change of reports required for authenticity. Writing a new narrative and stapling it to the old (D) would cause confusion as to which narrative was correct, especially if the forms became separated.

110. A

The bottom two ribs (called floating ribs) are not connected to the sternum. The other ribs are all connected to both the sternum and the spinal column.

111. B

While most behavioral calls are nonviolent, the potential for violence exists and warrants police presence. ALS units may have the ability to administer sedatives to violent patients, and might be included, but police would still be necessary. A second rescue or the fire department would only be necessary if more manpower was necessary to restrain the patient, if indicated.

112. C

Either 1 or 2 points is given for each of the five elements of the APGAR score, for a maximum of 10.

113. C

The normal range for blood glucose is 80–120. Low blood sugar or (C) is the correct answer. (A) is a condition where there is an excessive amount of sugar in the blood. (B) is a condition resulting from not enough insulin in the body, so ketones are produced, which turns the blood acidic.

114. A

Victims of sexual assault might prefer to share sensitive information with an EMT of their own gender. Police officers and rape crisis counselors are important in the follow-up treatment of these victims, as are registered nurses, but initial prehospital care should be done by an EMT, preferably one of the same gender.

115. C

Buccal (C) is a word relating to the cheek. While both (A) and (B) are located in the mouth, they are not specific to the cheek. (D) describes an area in the ear canal.

116. D

The most common EMS trauma call is for motor vehicle accidents.

117. B

Numerous studies have shown that survivability increases dramatically if a patient with severe trauma can have surgical intervention within the "golden hour," or 60 minutes.

118. D

The average adult human has 5–6 liters of blood.

119. B

A high temperature is the most frequent cause of pediatric seizures, followed by epilepsy, poisoning, and drug exposure to the fetus while in the mother's uterus.

120. A

Look at the presentation of the bleeding. While it does state that the bleeding is profuse, it also states that the bleeding is a steady flow and not spurting. Steady flow indicates a venous bleed, so a hemostatic agent (A) is appropriate to staunch the blood flow: it doesn't have the potential tissue damage of a tourniquet and it has more stopping power than just a pressure bandage. If the blood were pressurized and spurting, that would indicate a possible arterial bleed, which would require a tourniquet (B) without delay. (If your service does not carry hemostatic agents, then a tourniquet can be used, but it is less preferred.)

121. B

Since neonates and infants are nose-breathers, upper respiratory infections cause mucus buildup, which causes difficulty breathing in that population. Foreign bodies and birth defects can also cause dyspnea, but mucus is the most common cause. Sudden Infant Death Syndrome (SIDS) refers to a condition where a previously healthy infant is found dead with no explicable cause.

122. C

As EMTs work in all types of situations outside of a consistently clean environment that is the hospital, sterility is a big consideration. Non-sterile equipment or dressings can introduce bacteria into the patient's bloodstream, which could have serious consequences later. The most important feature of a dressing is that it come in a unopened package. Size and shape are important, too, but less important than sterility. Elasticity is not a factor unless specifically aiming for a compression type of bandage.

123. C

A patient may always change his or her mind, even after signing a refusal. When a patient refuses treatment or transport, all options must be explained as well as the possible medical consequences. The signature of the patient on the refusal form should be witnessed by a disinterested third party to attest to the facts of the refusal.

124. D

Trendelenburg position, the raising of the feet above the head, retaining body heat, and administration of oxygen are all treatments for shock. Fowler position is seated upright and is not indicated for treatment of hypovolemia.

125. C

Bruising is a type of closed wound; the skin is not open to the outside. Abrasions, incisions, and lacerations are all types of open wounds.

126. A

NTG (nitroglycerin) is a potent vasodilator, which accounts for its effectiveness in relieving chest pain caused by reduced blood flow in the carotid arteries. It consequently may lead to lowered blood pressure, or hypotension.

127. B

A wound in the neck that may leak air into the body should be dressed with an occlusive dressing to keep air from entering and contributing to a pneumothorax. Wounds to the genitals, head, and abdomen may be dressed with ordinary dressings.

128. B

By the rule of nines, each arm is 9% of body surface, so both arms would be a total of 18%.

129. C

Second-degree, or partial-thickness, burns are critical if they involve an entire body part. Normally a second-degree burn would be considered critical only if it involved more than 30% of body area.

130. A

Naloxone is a drug used for opioid overdoses, of which heroin is one. The total dosage given the IN route is 2 mg, making (A) the correct answer. LSD is not an opioid and NSAID stands for non-steroidal anti-inflammatory drug, of which ibuprofen would be one.

131. B

No matter the type of splint you use, the splint must be secured above and below the injury site (B) for full immobilization. By securing above and below the injury, you are securing the entire bone to limit additional movement. (Never secure a splint directly over a joint, as that could put tension on the ligaments/tendons and limit proper anatomical movement.) You would not splint over the injury, as that would be painful for the patient.

132. B

If a fracture occludes the artery feeding the distal portion of the extremity, then the cells will die and amputation becomes a real possibility. The goal in realigning the bone is to restore circulation to the extremity. The other fractures should be splinted as they are found.

133. B

SAMPLE stands for Signs and symptoms, Allergies, Medications, Past history, Last oral intake, and Events leading up to the situation.

134. B

The epiglottis is higher in the airway of an infant, an important anatomical difference.

135. D

Cervical spine injury should be considered in all trauma situations unless you can definitely rule it out. Neck pain brought about by sleeping also calls for immobilization until damage to the spinal cord can be ruled out.

136. D

(A), (B), and (C) are all necessary to the narrative, both to document what the EMT assessed about the patient for legal purposes and to assist the receiving physician in making his or her diagnosis.

137. B

The foaming of a wound to the chest indicates that the pleural cavity has been compromised; as the air pressure builds in the pleural space, the lung will not be able to expand normally. This condition is referred to as a pneumothorax.

138. B

Abdominal wounds are at a high risk for infection if the contents of the gastrointestinal tract spill into the abdominal compartment, especially if the wound is open and exposed to the air/bacteria. Hypertension and sudden cardiac death are always a possibility in serious injuries, as is peritonitis, but the best answer is infection (B).

139. C

Neonates are aged from birth to 4 weeks, infants from 4 weeks to 1 year, toddlers from 1 to 3 years, preschoolers from 3 to 6 years, school-age children from 6 to 10 years, and adolescents from 11 to 21 years of age.

140. D

A tourniquet once applied should never be released in the field since serious shock may develop; therefore, it should only be released once the patient is in the hospital and bleeding may be controlled surgically.

141. C

Four-point restraints require that each limb be restrained. The patient should always be supine so you can intervene immediately, should that become necessary for another medical condition such as cardiac arrest. Patients should never be restrained face down or prone, as that causes pressure on the diaphragm, which may lead to apnea and sudden death (and would not be apparent if the patient were face down). Likewise, the patient should never be made to lie on his restrained limbs due to the risk of impaired circulation in the extremities. Handcuffs are not approved EMS restraints and should be used only by authorized and trained police officers.

142. D

In order to properly immobilize a fractured hip, the patient must be secured to a long backboard. The other splints would not do this.

143. D

A lacerated artery will bleed more readily due to the higher pressure in the arteries, as well as due to the pulsing action that makes clotting more difficult. Arterioles are smaller arteries and will clot more readily than a larger vessel, and veins and capillaries flow at lower pressures that facilitate clotting.

144. B

Aspirin is given for chest pain due to its anticlotting action and is listed in most state protocols following the American Heart Association™ guidelines. Aspirin is also indicated for headache and other pain, but not usually in the emergency setting.

145. C

The police may obtain a copy of the report if they either get permission from the patient or obtain a search warrant from a judge or magistrate. Note the use of the qualifying word *routinely* in the question.

146. B

The correct answer is (B), which is the Emergency Response Guide. (A) is used to measure brain waves, while (D) measures heart rhythms. (C) stands for ear, nose, and throat.

147. A

A first pregnancy will normally have a longer labor and delivery time than the subsequent pregnancies.

148. B

The ambulance should be used to protect the scene in order to avoid injury to the EMTs and the patients.

149. A

The second stage of labor occurs when the baby is forced out of the uterus by the contractions down into the mother's vagina and ends with the birth of the baby. The first stage of labor is from the expulsion of the mucus plug through the baby's expulsion from the uterus, and the third stage follows the birth of the baby when the placenta is delivered.

150. C

Implied consent means that in the case of a patient who cannot give consent, such as an individual who is unconscious, consent for treatment is implied and constitutes what the average person would want under similar circumstances.

Your Practice Test Score

The practice test in this book is designed to give you experience answering multiple-choice questions about EMT content.

- Recall that the EMT Exam is a CAT, a computer-based test that adapts to your ability. At the start of the exam, the computer assumes you have average aptitude and gives you a "medium-difficulty" question. After each question that you answer correctly, the computer increases its estimate of your ability and gives you a more difficult question. And vice versa: if you answer a question incorrectly, you are given an easier question.

- Your score on the real exam is determined by an algorithm that calculates your ability level based not just on what you got right or wrong, but also on the difficulty level of the questions you answered.

- As a result, the **paper and pencil practice test here can provide only limited feedback on scoring**.

Additionally, **there is no actual point score on the exam**. Instead, the NREMT governing body aims for a 95% confidence rate; in other words, as a result of you answering questions right or wrong, your exam will be "scored" based on whether there is 95% confidence that you have met minimal entry-level competency.

Therefore, to "score" your practice exam, calculate the percentage of questions you answered correctly:

1. Number of questions right divided by 150 = **decimal answer**
2. Take decimal answer × 100 = **percentage**
   - Example: 120/150 = 0.8 ⟶ 0.8 × 100 = 80%
   - Example: 75/150 = 0.5 ⟶ 0.5 × 100 = 50%

Your Score	Now What?
80% or better	You have a good understanding of essential EMT content and are able to use the knowledge and thinking skills required to answer exam-style questions. Consider scheduling your NR cognitive exam, and remember to study a little bit every day until Test Day to keep it fresh in your mind.
60–79%	You have areas of EMT content that need further review, and/or you may need continued work to master the knowledge and thinking skills required to be successful on the cognitive exam. If you schedule your cognitive exam now, you may or may not pass it. Keep in mind that you are charged an exam fee for every attempt.
59% or less	You need concentrated study of EMT content and continued practice utilizing the knowledge and thinking skills required to be successful on the cognitive exam. It is suggested that you hold off on scheduling your cognitive exam at this time. Dedicate more time to studying the basics. Review your textbook, and then go back through these chapters and practice questions.

EMT-Basic Resources

GLOSSARY

A

Abandonment: failure to properly treat an ill or injured person who is in need of emergency medical care

Abdominal quadrants: the four sections of the abdomen, using the umbilicus (navel) as the focal point: upper left, upper right, lower left, lower right

Abrasion: type of wound in which the epidermis is scraped by an object, causing little blood loss but with increased danger of infection due to the amount of dermis exposed

Activated charcoal: charcoal in liquid suspension used to absorb ingested poisons

Active rewarming: use of heat packs and heated fluids to rewarm a hypothermic patient

Acute: immediate

Adolescent: pediatric patient age 11–21

Advance directive: medical decisions made by a patient or caregiver in advance, usually in the form of do-not-resuscitate orders

Afterbirth: placenta and fetal membranes that are expelled from the mother following delivery of a baby

Allergic reaction: severe and unusual response of the body to a foreign substance

Altered mental status: inappropriate response to normal stimuli, i.e., being responsive only to voice, only to pain, or being unconscious; also used to describe abnormal behavior

Alveoli: sacs in the lung in which oxygen is exchanged for carbon dioxide in the red blood cells

Amniotic sac: bag of fluid that surrounds and protects the fetus during pregnancy; usually ruptures prior to delivery

Amputation: complete separation of a body part from the body

Anaphylaxis: consequence of an allergic reaction, where the body responds with swelling of respiratory tissues and shock

Aorta: large artery at the top of the heart carrying blood to all major arteries

Apnea: lack of breathing, absence of respiratory activity

Arterioles: vessels that connect the arteries to the capillaries

Arteriosclerosis (or hardening of the arteries): disease process in which the arteries lose elasticity as they become rigid

Arteries: vessels that carry oxygenated blood from the aorta to the arterioles

Aspiration: inhaling of foreign substances into the trachea, bronchial tree, and lungs

Asystole: cardiac standstill, lack of electrical activity in the heart muscle

Atria: the two uppermost chambers of the heart

Aura: visual, auditory, olfactory, or other sense of an impending seizure

Auscultation: listening for sounds within the body, usually with a stethoscope

Automated external defibrillator (AED): device that attempts to overcome certain cardiac dysrhythmias with an electrical countershock; operates by interpreting the cardiac rhythm and responding appropriately without the need for operator interpretation

AVPU: acronym used for determining level of consciousness: Alert, responsive to Verbal, responsive to Pain, Unresponsive

Avulsion: forcible tearing away of tissue as a result of blunt-force trauma

B

Bag-valve mask: respiratory device used to manually support respirations in cases of respiratory distress or apnea

Bandage: cloth used to secure a sterile dressing to a wound

Baseline vital signs: vital signs taken first and used to track a patient's improvement or decline

Battle sign: ecchymosis behind the ears that suggests a basilar skull fracture

Behavioral emergency: emergency medical call in which the patient's actions are bizarre and inappropriate

Bilateral: referring to both the right and left sides of the body

Bipolar disorder: psychiatric condition in which a patient alternates between extremes of euphoria and depression; extremes may last from a few minutes to several months

Blood pressure: pressure (in millimeters of mercury) of the blood flow through the arteries

Blood pressure cuff (sphygmomanometer): device used to measure blood pressure by applying pressure to an artery

Body substance isolation (BSI): important act of protection of an EMT from airborne and bloodborne pathogens by the use of personal protective equipment (PPE)

Brachial artery: large artery in the upper arm that feeds the entire extremity

Bradycardia: heart rate slower than 60 beats per minute

Bradypnea: respiratory rate slower than eight respirations per minute

Breech birth: presentation of any part of a fetus other than the head during delivery

Bronchi: two tubes that connect the trachea to the bronchioles

Bronchioles: smaller tubes that connect the bronchi to the alveoli

Burn sheet: large sterile dressing used to cover burn injuries

C

Capillaries: small blood vessels in which oxygen is given off to the cells for metabolism and waste products are collected

Capillary refill: diagnostic sign in which the nail bed is blanched by applying pressure and the time for it to return to normal color is measured, normally less than 2 seconds

Cardiac arrest: condition caused by the heart's failure to pump blood

Carotid arteries: large arteries that feed the brain

Central nervous system (CNS): brain and spinal cord

Cerebrovascular accident (CVA) (stroke): ischemia in the brain caused by either a cerebral hemorrhage or thrombus

Chief complaint: illness or injury for which the emergency medical system was activated

Chronic obstructive pulmonary disease (COPD): degeneration of the alveoli by disease processes causing progressive dyspnea; examples are emphysema and chronic bronchitis

Chronic: long-term gradual process

Conduction: method of heat transfer in which heat is transferred by direct contact between bodies

Congestive heart failure (CHF): condition of dyspnea in which fluid backs up into the lungs caused by failure of the heart's pumping action

Contraindications: situations in which a drug or protocol should not be used

Contusion: hemorrhage that occurs beneath the skin; bruising

Convection: method of heat transfer from the body caused by air passing over it

Convulsion: seizure activity of the body

Critical incident stress debriefing (CISD): discussion of a stressful incident, with the goal of allowing an EMT to deal with the emotions encountered and move on

Crowning: appearance of the top of the baby's head in the birth canal during delivery

Cushing reflex: increased blood pressure, decreased heart rate, and respiratory changes caused by hypoxia in the brain; indicative of severe head injury

Cyanosis: bluish-gray color indicative of poor circulatory perfusion

D

Decerebrate posturing: when a patient extends arms outward and arches the back; indicates a more severe head injury

Decorticate posturing: when a patient flexes arms inward and arches the back; indicates a severe head injury

Defibrillation: correction of cardiac fibrillation by electrical countershock

Dementia: abnormal behavior brought about by disease of the brain

Dermis: intermediate layer of skin between the epidermis and fatty tissue or muscle

Diabetes: disease of the pancreas that inhibits the body's ability to process sugars

Diastolic blood pressure: pressure in the arteries while the heart is at rest

Dressing: sterile pad placed directly on a wound

Drowning: death caused by suffocation in water

Drug: any chemical introduced into the body (prescribed or otherwise) that causes a change in how the body functions or responds

Dyspnea: difficulty breathing

E

Ecchymosis: black-and-blue discoloration caused by subcutaneous hemorrhage

Endocrine system: system of the body that produces hormones used in the metabolic process

Epidermis: top layer of skin

Epidural: layer between the skull and the dura mater of the brain and spine

Epilepsy (seizure disorder): disease of the brain that causes seizures

Epinephrine: natural hormone that helps the body regulate multiple processes; also a medication used for heart irregularities and anaphylaxis

Epistaxis: bleeding from the nose

Esophagus: body's tubular passage from the pharynx to the stomach

Evisceration: traumatic opening of the abdominal cavity in which the intestines protrude to the outside

Expressed consent: formal consent from a competent patient for treatment and/or transport

Extubation: removal of a breathing tube

F

Femoral artery: large artery in the upper leg that feeds the entire extremity

Femur: large bone of the upper leg

Fetus: child in the uterus before birth

Fibula: one of two bones in the lower leg

Flail segment: ≥2 ribs broken in ≥2 places

Fontanelle: soft spot in a baby's skull where bones have not yet fused together

Fowler position: position in which patient is sitting upright; normally best for conscious patients with dyspnea

French catheter: soft-suction catheter

Full-thickness burn (formerly known as third-degree burn): burn that extends through the epidermis and dermis to the tissues below

G

Glucose: form of sugar used by the body for fuel

Guarding: position in which a patient places the hands over the part of the body that is painful

H

Hard catheter: rigid-suction catheter

Hazardous material: any material that is dangerous to one's health or safety

Head-tilt, chin-lift: procedure in which the airway of a non-trauma patient is secured; one hand is placed on the patient's forehead and tilted back, while the other hand lifts the chin

Hives: itchy, red blotches on the skin associated with allergic reactions

Hot zone: in a hazardous-materials incident, the area that contains the hazardous material; only personnel in proper protective equipment should enter this zone

Hyper-: prefix meaning higher; more; faster

Hyperthermia: overheated, having a high temperature

Hypo-: prefix meaning lower; below; less; slower

Hypoglycemia: low blood sugar

Hypothermia: cold, having a low temperature

Hypovolemia: low blood volume

Hypoxia: low oxygen level

I

Immune response: body's response to a foreign invader

Implied consent: assumption that consent would be given for treatment/transport if the patient were conscious

Incident command system: system of command and control at a mass casualty or disaster scene

Indications: situations in which a drug or protocol should be followed

Infant: pediatric patient age 1–12 months

Ingestion: process in which an object is taken into the mouth and swallowed

Inhalation (inspiration): process in which an object is brought into the lungs through the nose and mouth

Initial assessment: first impression of a patient's condition after scene size-up

Injection: process in which a substance is introduced into the body by a needle

In-line stabilization: holding of the head and neck in a straight-line neutral position to minimize the danger of damaging the spinal cord during treatment and transport

Inspiration (inhalation): process by which an object is brought into the lungs through the nose and mouth

Insulin: hormone used by the body to metabolize sugars

Intercostal muscles: muscles between the ribs used in the breathing process

Intracranial pressure (ICP): pressure within the skull

Intubation: placement of a tube into the trachea to facilitate rescue breathing (not an EMT-Basic skill)

Intravenous (IV): into a vein (i.e., giving medication via this method)

J

Jaundice: yellowish appearance of the skin, commonly caused by diseases of the liver

Jaw-thrust maneuver: maneuver to open the airway of a trauma patient; head and neck are maintained in a neutral position while the jaw is lifted upward to open the airway

Joint: location where two bones meet

K

Kinetics: study of physical laws of motion (used for trauma assessment)

L

Labor: process through which a baby is born; begins when the mucus plug blocking the cervix is expelled and concludes with the delivery of the placenta

Laceration: wound in which the skin is opened by a cut or tear

Ligaments: bands of tissue that connect muscles, bones, and joints

Lungs: organs comprised of small air sacs in which oxygenated air is inhaled and passes into the blood, while carbon-dioxide waste is removed

M

Main stem bronchi: large tubes connecting the trachea to the lungs

Malaise: general feeling of illness

Mammalian diving reflex: body's response to sudden immersion into cold water, when vital systems reflexively shut down to preserve oxygen

Mantoux test: test for tuberculosis bacteria

Mass casualty incident (MCI): incident with one or more patients that the initial arriving unit can safely treat and transport

Mechanism of injury (MOI): manner in which an injury occurs

Meconium: waste product expelled by a distressed fetus during delivery

Medical control: the EMT's supervising medical professional(s)

Medical direction: protocols and practices given to EMTs by a physician

Medication: any substance introduced into a body to affect healing or alleviation of abnormal symptoms

Meninges: layers of tissue surrounding the brain and spinal cord

Metered-dose inhaler: device prescribed to patients to deliver a prescribed dosage of medication to be inhaled; often prescribed for asthma and other respiratory illnesses

Minor consent: permission obtained from a responsible adult for a minor child or incapacitated adult

Miscarriage: expulsion of a fetus and products of conception before the fetus is viable

N

Nasal cannula: oxygen delivery device that delivers 2–6 liters per minute into the nasopharynx

Nasogastric tube: tube inserted into the nose and down into the stomach to suction possible toxins and/or administer medication directly into the stomach

Nasopharyngeal airway: airway device inserted into the nose and nasopharynx

Nature of illness (NOI): signs and symptoms of patient's illness

Negligence: legally defined as failure to act as a reasonable and prudent person would under similar circumstances

Neonate: pediatric patient from age birth to 1 month

Nervous system: system of sensory and motor nerves that control the human body functions, both voluntary and involuntary

Neurogenic shock: type of shock brought about by damage to the central nervous system that causes vasodilation; results in hypovolemia

Neurological deficit: any lessening or absence of the body's nervous-system response

Nitroglycerin (NTG): medication used for chest pain that causes vasodilation, which increases oxygen flow to the heart

Non-rebreather mask: oxygen delivery device that delivers 10–15 liters per minute; the reservoir bag provides 100% oxygen to the patient

O

Obstetric: having to do with delivery or childbirth

Occlusive dressing: sterile covering that seals off the wound from air; dressings of impermeable material or impregnated with sterile petroleum jelly

Offline medical direction: written standard protocols from an EMS medical director

Ongoing assessment: continuous monitoring of a patient while en route to a receiving facility

Online medical direction: direct contact with a physician to obtain orders or consultation

Open fracture: a broken bone associated with an open wound

Oral airway: device that assists in holding the tongue clear of the airway and maintaining a clear passage through the oropharynx

Oral glucose: high concentration of sugar given orally to a conscious patient with hypoglycemia

Orbits: the openings in the skull for the eyeballs

Oropharyngeal airway: specific type of oral airway, shaped like the letter "J" and inserted into the mouth to hold the tongue down

Overdose: misuse of any substance by ingesting, inhaling, or absorbing more than needed

Oxygen: element used by the body for metabolism, constituting 21% of normal air; supplemental oxygen is often given to assist breathing and metabolism in times of illness/injury

Oxygen humidifier: bottle of sterile water placed in-line with oxygen flow to provide moisture and prevent drying out of the pharynx

P

Pallor: pale or abnormally light skin color

Palpation: feeling with the hands and fingers

Paradoxical motion: opposite motion from the norm; describes the effect when a flail segment moves in an opposite-to-normal direction during breathing

Paranoia: mental illness categorized by deep feelings of persecution

Paresthesia: loss of sensation or paralysis in an extremity

Partial-thickness burn (formerly known as second-degree burn): burn causing blisters that extends through the epidermis and dermis but not below

Passive rewarming: reheating of a hypothermic patient by raising the ambient temperature, removing cold and wet clothing, and applying blankets to utilize the patient's own body heat

Patent airway: open, secure airway

Pathogens: substances that cause disease

Patient assessment: medical examination to determine mechanisms of injury and manner of illnesses

Perfusion: physiology of delivery of oxygen to the cells for the metabolic process

Peritonitis: infection of the abdominal cavity

Personal protective equipment (PPE): any device used by an EMT to protect against airborne and bloodborne pathogens

Pharynx: area between the mouth and the epiglottis, in which the trachea and esophagus separate

Phobia: mental illness manifesting itself in irrational fears

Physiology: study of the body's systems and functions

Placenta: organ that feeds the fetus during pregnancy; attaches to the wall of the uterus and is discharged after delivery of the fetus

Plasma: liquid component of blood

Platelets: component of blood that produces the clotting effect

Pleural space: space between the outer walls of the lungs

Pneumothorax: collapse of the lung caused by air buildup in the chest

Pocket mask: device for providing artificial ventilation by allowing an EMT to utilize his own exhalation to inflate a victim's lungs

Poison: any substance that inhibits the body's normal processes

Positive pressure ventilation: type of ventilation where lungs are inflated by a device that forces in air; may be a mechanical ventilator, pocket mask, or a bag-valve mask

Postictal state: state of unconsciousness following a seizure

Prehospital care report (PCR): summary of observations and interactions between the emergency medical service and a patient; this document is left with the receiving facility to become a permanent part of the patient's record

Premature infant: infant who is delivered before 36 weeks of gestation

Preschooler: pediatric patient age 3–6 years

Pressure point: place in which an artery crosses a bone and pressure can reduce hemorrhage

Primary triage: in an MCI, the first categorization of degree of injury, with the primary goal of identifying the most severely injured patients and prioritizing them for treatment and transport

Prolapsed cord: abnormal delivery situation in which the umbilical cord presents from the birth canal before the fetus

Prone: position of a body face down

Protocols: series of directives approved by a medical director for EMS to follow in given situations

Pulmonary edema: fluid in the lungs

Pulmonary embolism: blockage in the circulatory system of the lungs caused by a clot or bubble of air

Pulse: movement of blood through the arteries caused by contraction of the left ventricle

Pulse oximetry: measurement of oxygen perfusion, measured by the infrared signature of red blood cells

Pulse pressure: difference between the systolic and diastolic blood pressure

Pulseless electrical activity (PEA): random electrical activity of the heart that fails to produce a pulse

R

Raccoon sign: ecchymosis around the eyes, which may be symptomatic of a basilar skull fracture

Radiation: method of heat transfer in which there is no direct contact between bodies

Rapid extrication: method of removal of a patient from a hazardous situation without using normal precautions due to imminent danger

Rapid medical assessment: method of assessing an unconscious patient from head to toe to ascertain medical problems and to check for injuries

Rapid trauma assessment: method of assessing an unconscious patient from head to toe to check for injuries if there is a substantial mechanism of injury

Reasonable force: legal definition used to describe the minimum amount of force needed to restrain a patient in order to prevent injury to the patient or others

Red blood cells: component of the blood that carries oxygen to the cells

Repeaters: radios that amplify a radio signal and enable it to carry longer distances

Respiration: inhaling oxygen into the lungs for the metabolic process

Respiratory arrest: absence of spontaneous respirations

Respiratory failure: inability of the body to bring in adequate oxygen for the metabolic process

Retractions: depressions in the neck and chest cavity indicating use of the accessory muscles for respirations; indicative of respiratory distress

Rigid catheter (tonsil-tip suction): hard plastic suction device

Route: manner of drug delivery: oral, intravenous (IV), sublingual, buccal, intramuscular, intraosseous, or endotracheal

Rule of nines: method for rapidly determining the extent of a burn injury; divides body surface area of an adult body into 11 zones of 9% each

S

SAMPLE: diagnostic mnemonic that stands for: Signs and Symptoms, Allergies, Medications, Pertinent history, Last oral intake, and Events leading to current illness or injury

Scene safety: primary concern of an arriving EMT that the situation into which he or she is arriving is as hazard-free as possible

Scene size-up: quick assessment of a scene upon arrival to determine scene safety, number of victims, and need for additional or special units

Schizophrenia: mental illness categorized by delusions, blunted affect, thought disorders, and sometimes catatonia

School age: pediatric patient age 6–12

Scope of practice: medical procedures that are legally permitted to any individual dependent on level of licensure and training

Secondary triage: in an MCI, triage of a specific patient's condition to determine treatment and transport

Seizure: alteration in neurologic function that can include behavioral changes, muscle tremors, and loss of consciousness

Semi-Fowler position: position in which patient is sitting at a 45° angle; normally the best position for conscious patients with mild dyspnea and cardiac symptoms

Shock: situation in which cells are not properly oxygenated due to loss of blood, also known as hypoperfusion syndrome

Side effects: effects of any drug or procedure other than its intended effect

Signs: objective measurements of a body's response to illness and/or injury

Snoring: sound made by a partial obstruction of the upper airway

Soft catheter (French catheter): suction device of soft plastic

Sphygmomanometer (blood pressure cuff): device used to measure blood pressure by applying pressure to an artery

Spinal column: bony structure of the back that protects the spinal cord

Spinal cord: series of nerves leading from the base of the brain that carry impulses to the muscles and sensory information back to the brain

Spinal shock: shock caused by injury to the spinal cord that affects its ability to transmit the necessary nerve impulses for normal perfusion

Splint: any device that immobilizes a bone or joint

Spontaneous abortion (miscarriage): any termination of pregnancy that occurs before a fetus is able to remain viable

Staging sector: section where units are deployed to remain ready to respond to specific assignments at a mass casualty incident

Standard of care: level of medical treatment that is normal and expected for a given situation

Standing orders: procedures that medical control deems suitable for the EMT to perform under given situations without the need to contact medical control (see offline medical direction)

Status epilepticus: seizures lasting longer than a few minutes or multiple seizures that occur without an intervening period of lucidity

Sterile: objects free from pathogens

Stoma: opening in the neck bypassing the pharynx to enable breathing

Stridor: high-pitched wheezing sound indicating upper airway swelling or obstruction

Stroke (cerebrovascular accident [CVA]): brain damage caused by a clot or hemorrhage in the cerebrum or cerebellum

Subarachnoid hemorrhage: bleeding between the brain and the arachnoid membrane

Subcutaneous layer: layer of tissue directly below the skin

Subdural hematoma: bleeding beneath the dura, or outer covering of the brain

Sucking chest wound: open wound that extends into the lung cavity, causing deflation of the lung (pneumothorax)

Sudden infant death syndrome (SIDS): medical condition affecting infants who die suddenly and without any explanation

Suicide: the taking of one's own life

Superficial burn: (formerly known as first-degree burn): burn that involves only the epidermis; common example is a sunburn

Supine hypotensive syndrome: condition seen in late pregnancy, where the weight of the fetus impairs the return circulation of blood and causes low blood pressure and inadequate perfusion

Supply sector: MCI location where supplies are brought for units to restock

Syncope: brief period of loss of consciousness

Systolic blood pressure: pressure in the arteries while the ventricles contract

T

Tachycardia: sustained fast heart rate in excess of 100 beats per minute

Tachypnea: sustained fast respiratory rate in excess of 20 breaths per minute

Tension pneumothorax: collapse of a lung, where the organs in the chest begin to shift into the space vacated by the collapsed lung

Tidal volume: amount of air inhaled in a normal respiratory effort

Toddler: pediatric patient age 1–3 years

Toxin: substance that poisons the body

Trachea: tube connecting the mouth and nose to the lungs

Tracheostomy: surgical opening in the neck that allows a patient with an occluded airway to breathe

Transient ischemic attack (TIA): condition that causes temporary stroke-like symptoms (up to 24 hours), caused by spasms of the arteries in the brain

Transportation sector: in an MCI, the area in which patients are transported to appropriate medical facilities

Trauma: sudden injury caused by the application of external forces to a human body

Treatment sector: in an MCI, the area in which patients are given initial treatment before transport

Trendelenburg position: patient lies face upward on a tilted table or bed with pelvis higher than the head

Triage: process of determining the severity of injuries in order to best utilize available resources; normally there are four groups: red for critical patients, yellow for serious patients, green for slightly injured ambulatory patients, and black for patients who are dead or mortally wounded

Triage sector: in an MCI, the area in which triage occurs and is controlled; initial triage occurs where the patient is found

Triage tag: tag that allows the EMT to mark the patient's status and initial impressions; also used to account for patients as they pass through the various sectors in an MCI

Tripod position: position often assumed by patients in severe respiratory distress, i.e., seated with arms to the side and rotated forward to facilitate breathing

U

Umbilical cord: vessel that connects a fetus to the placenta in utero

Umbilicus: the navel, i.e., area where the umbilical cord is connected to fetus's abdomen

Urgent move: situation in which a patient is moved quickly due to the seriousness of the condition or immediate danger of further injury

Uterus: female organ which harbors a fetus during pregnancy

V

Vein: blood vessel that carries blood toward the heart

Venae cavae: main veins leading directly into the heart

Ventilation: passage of air into and out of the lungs

Ventricles: the two lower chambers of the heart

Ventricular fibrillation (V-Fib): cardiac condition in which the heart muscles vibrate rather than contract, resulting in collapse of circulation

Ventricular tachycardia (V-Tach): rapid heartbeat that frequently fails to produce a pulse and thus fails to produce perfusion

Venules: small blood vessels leading from the capillaries to the veins

Vital signs: assessments of an ill or injured patient that are objectively measured, including blood pressure, heart rate, respiratory rate, pupil response, and oxygen saturation

Voluntary guarding: contractions of the abdominal wall, as a response to pain or injury

W

Warm zone: in a hazardous-material incident, the area adjacent to the hot zone where injured patients are moved so that they can receive decontamination, triage, and treatment

Water chill: increase in loss of body heat due to presence of water

White blood cells: component of the blood that combats infection in the body

Wind chill: increase in loss of body heat due to wind speed

Withdrawal: body's response to the cessation of use of alcohol or narcotic substances

X

Xiphoid process: bony inferior tip of the sternum

State EMS Certification Links

Alabama

Office of Emergency Medical Services and Trauma
http://www.adph.org/ems

Alaska

Emergency Medical Services
http://www.chems.alaska.gov/EMS/default.htm

Arizona

Bureau of Emergency Medical Services and Trauma System
http://www.azdhs.gov/bems

Arkansas

Emergency Medical Services and Trauma Systems
https://www.healthy.arkansas.gov/programs-services/topics/ems-resources

California

Emergency Medical Services Authority
http://www.emsa.ca.gov

Colorado

Emergency Medical and Trauma Services
http://www.cdphe.state.co.us/em/index.html

Connecticut

Emergency Medical Services
http://www.ct.gov/dph/cwp/view.asp?a=3127&q=387362

District of Columbia

Fire and Emergency Medical Services
https://fems.dc.gov

Delaware

Emergency Medical Services
https://www.dhss.delaware.gov/dph/ems/paramediceducation.html

Florida

Bureau of Emergency Medical Services
http://www.floridahealth.gov/licensing-and-regulation/emt-paramedics/index.html

Georgia

Emergency Medical Services
http://ems.ga.gov/

Hawaii

Emergency Medical Services & Injury Prevention System Branch
https://health.hawaii.gov/ems/home/certification-and-licensure-for-ems-providers-and-personnel/

Idaho

Emergency Medical Services
https://www.idahoemslicense.net/lms/public/portal#/login

Illinois

Emergency Medical Systems and Highway Safety
http://www.idph.state.il.us/ems/index.htm

Indiana

Emergency Medical Services
https://www.in.gov/dhs/4142.htm

Iowa

Bureau of Emergency Medical Services
https://idph.iowa.gov/BETS/EMS

Kansas

Board of Emergency Medical Services
http://www.ksbems.org

Kentucky

Board of Emergency Medical Services
http://kbems.kctcs.edu/index.html

Louisiana

Emergency Medical Services
http://ldh.la.gov/index.cfm/page/759

Maine

Maine Emergency Medical Services
http://www.state.me.us/dps/ems

Maryland

Institute for Emergency Medical Services Systems
https://www.miemsslicense.com/lms/public/portal#/login

Massachusetts

Office of Emergency Medical Services
http://www.mass.gov/dph/oems

Michigan

Emergency Medical Services
http://www.michigan.gov/ems

Minnesota

Emergency Medical Services Regulatory Board
http://www.emsrb.state.mn.us

Mississippi

Emergency Medical Services
http://www.ems.doh.ms.gov/ems/index.html

Missouri

Emergency Medical Services
https://health.mo.gov/safety/ems/licensing.php

Montana

EMS & Trauma Systems
https://dphhs.mt.gov/publichealth/emsts

Nebraska

Emergency Medical Services
http://dhhs.ne.gov/Pages/EHS-EMS-Licensing.aspx

Nevada

Emergency Medical Services
http://dpbh.nv.gov/Reg/EMS/dta/Licensing/Emergency_Medical_System_(EMS)_-_Licensing/

New Hampshire

Bureau of Emergency Medical Services
https://www.nh.gov/safety/divisions/fstems/ems/index.html

New Jersey

Office of Emergency Medical Services
http://www.state.nj.us/health/ems/index.shtml

New Mexico

Emergency Medical Services Bureau
http://www.nmems.org

New York

Bureau of Emergency Medical Services
http://www.health.state.ny.us/nysdoh/ems/main.htm

North Carolina

Office of Emergency Medical Services
http://facility-services.state.nc.us/EMS/ems.htm

North Dakota

Division of Emergency Medical Services and Trauma
http://www.ndhealth.gov/EMS/

Ohio

Division of Emergency Medical Services
http://www.ems.ohio.gov

Oklahoma

Emergency Medical Services Division
http://www.ok.gov/health/Protective_Health/Emergency_Medical_Services/

Oregon

Emergency Medical Services and Trauma Systems
*https://www.oregon.gov/oha/ph/providerpartnerresources/emstraumasystems/
emstrainingcertification/Pages/index.aspx*

Pennsylvania

Emergency Medical Services
https://www.health.pa.gov/topics/EMS/Pages/FAQ.aspx

Rhode Island

Division of Emergency Medical Services
https://health.ri.gov/licenses/detail.php?id=284

South Carolina

Emergency Medical Services
https://www.scdhec.gov/health-professionals/ems-training-protocols-requirements

South Dakota

Office of Emergency Medical Services
http://dps.sd.gov/emergency_services/emergency_medical_services/default.aspx

Tennessee

Emergency Medical Services
*https://www.tn.gov/health/health-program-areas/health-professional-boards/ems-board/
ems-board/licensure.html*

Texas

Emergency Medical Services
http://www.dshs.state.tx.us/emstraumasystems/emsdirectory.shtm

Utah

Bureau of Emergency Medical Services
http://health.utah.gov/ems

Vermont

Emergency Medical Services
http://healthvermont.gov/hc/ems/ems_index.aspx

Virginia

Office of Emergency Medical Services
https://www.vdh.virginia.gov/emergency-medical-services/education-certification/

Washington

Office of Emergency Medical Services and Trauma System
https://www.doh.wa.gov/ForPublicHealthandHealthcareProviders/EmergencyMedicalServices EMSSystems/EMSProviderCertification

West Virginia

Office of Emergency Medical Services
http://www.wvoems.org

Wisconsin

Emergency Medical Services
http://www.dhs.wisconsin.gov/ems/licensing/index.htm

Wyoming

Emergency Medical Services
https://health.wyo.gov/publichealth/ems/ems-program-2/ems-licensure/

Answer Key for Test Yourself Questions

Test Yourself 2.1

While the parents are not on scene to give consent, an EMS professional acting under *in loco parentis* would still be able to render care. However, an attempt must be made to reach the parents/guardians in order to, at a minimum, notify them of the child's transport, but also to gain consent. This should also be fully documented in your patient care report as well as the number of times contact was attempted and/or made. It is also a good practice to get the name of a parent/guardian in order to document that in your PCR.

As unusual as it may sound, certain parents/guardians may not want their children transported, and that is their right, but efforts must be made to explain the necessity (or not) of treatment so informed consent can be obtained.

Test Yourself 3.1

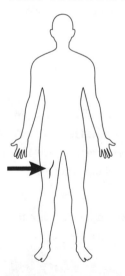

Test Yourself 4.1

O: I was lifting weights and all of a sudden, I felt a sharp pain.

P: If I raise my left arm, it gets a lot worse. I've never had anything like this before.

Q: I felt a sharp pain right here [points to left chest superior to his left nipple]. It feels like a tearing sensation.

R: The pain doesn't move.

S: I would rate it about 6 on a scale of 1 to 10.

T: The pain started right after I finished exercising an hour ago. It's the first time this has happened.

His answers would point toward an injury to the pectoral muscle during his exercising, rather than to another condition, such as a heart attack.

Test Yourself 4.2

RTS score would be 11. The only point lost on the RTS is from the low blood pressure.

Test Yourself 4.3

This is a challenging question and it relies both on hard data (e.g., blood sugar level, GCS) and on the patient's presentation in general. As he is able to answer your questions despite the slurred words and is cooperative with your commands and requests, he is not necessarily "altered." Your best bet is to consult medical command and request permission to administer more glucose (or have the patient speak to a doctor) or to request that ALS come for further evaluation.

This is one of those situations that comes down to ethical and legal critical decision making. Do you think he is a danger to himself or others? Could having him sign a refusal at this point be a legal minefield? If he is given more medication, will the issue resolve itself?

Test Yourself 5.1

You would use a head-tilt, chin-lift maneuver since you can rule out cervical trauma, as her fainting episode happened right in front of you. If she struck her head on the ground, you could potentially use the jaw thrust. As she has facial and specifically nasal trauma, you would use an OPA. Finally, you would use a hard-tipped suction catheter (Yankauer) tip, as her mouth is easily opened.

Test Yourself 5.2

This type of question requires the EMT to think critically.. The patient is normally on oxygen at 2 lpm on a daily basis but for whatever reason, his oxygen is not on currently. He is not in any obvious respiratory distress and his SpO2 levels are near the low end of "normal" at 94%. The most correct answer is that if he is normally on oxygen, the EMT should continue this therapy, as perhaps without the oxygen the patient could desaturate.

However, if the patient is not presenting with respiratory difficulty, the EMT may elect not to use the oxygen at first and simply monitor the oxygen level closely.

Test Yourself 7.1

All the burns are anterior so we are working with half of each arm. Remember that the forearm is the lower half of the arm, below the elbow. If each arm is worth anteriorly 4.5%, then half of the arm for the forearm and hand would be 2.25%. Since it is both forearms and hands, this would equal 4.5%.

The chest in total is worth 9%. So if only half of the chest is burned such as our scenario with the "upper chest," this is 4.5%. So add 4.5 + 4.5 = 9% total burned.